Hallux Valgus Deformity and Treatment: A Three-Dimensional Approach

Editor

WOO-CHUN LEE

FOOT AND ANKLE CLINICS

www.foot.theclinics.com

Consulting Editor
MARK S. MYERSON

June 2018 • Volume 23 • Number 2

ELSEVIER

1600 John F. Kennedy Boulevard • Suite 1800 • Philadelphia, Pennsylvania, 19103-2899

http://www.theclinics.com

FOOT AND ANKLE CLINICS Volume 23, Number 2
June 2018 ISSN 1083-7515, ISBN-13: 978-0-323-61054-4

Editor: Lauren Boyle
Developmental Editor: Meredith Madeira

Foot and Ankle Clinics (ISSN 1083-7515) is published quarterly by Elsevier, Inc., 360 Park Avenue South, New York, NY 10010-1710. Months of issue are March, June, September, and December. Periodicals postage paid at New York, NY, and additional mailing offices. Subscription price per year is $326.00 (US individuals), $519.00 (US institutions), $100.00 (US students), $367.00 (Canadian individuals), $623.00 (Canadian institutions), $215.00 (Canadian students), $460.00 (international individuals), $623.00 (international institutions), and $215.00 (international students). To receive student/resident rate, orders must be accompanied by name of affiliated institution, date of term, and the *signature* of program/residency coordinator on institution letterhead. Orders will be billed at individual rate until proof of status is received. Foreign air speed delivery is included in all *Clinics* subscription prices. All prices are subject to change without notice. **POSTMASTER:** Send address changes to *Foot and Ankle Clinics*, Elsevier Health Sciences Division, Subscription Customer Service, 3251 Riverport Lane, Maryland Heights, MO 63043. **Customer Service: 1-800-654-2452 (US and Canada). From outside of the United States and Canada, call 314-447-8871. Fax: 314-447-8029. E-mail: JournalsCustomerService-usa@ elsevier.com (for print support); JournalsOnlineSupport-usa@elsevier.com (for online support).**

Reprints. For copies of 100 or more, of articles in this publication, please contact the Commercial Reprints Department, Elsevier Inc., 360 Park Avenue South, New York, NY 10010-1710. Tel.: 212-633-3874; Fax: 212-633-3820; E-mail: reprints@elsevier.com.

Contributors

CONSULTING EDITOR

MARK S. MYERSON, MD
Medical Director, The Foot and Ankle Association, Inc, Baltimore, Maryland, USA

EDITOR

WOO-CHUN LEE, MD
Seoul Foot and Ankle Center, Dubalo Orthopaedic Clinic, Seoul, Korea

AUTHORS

AMIETHAB A. AIYER, MD
Assistant Professor, Department of Orthopaedic Surgery, University of Miami, Miami, Florida, USA

NAJI AL-KHUDAIRI, MBBS, BSc
Royal National Orthopaedic Hospital, London, United Kingdom

STEVEN BLACKWOOD, MD
Fellow, Orthopaedic Associates of Michigan, Grand Rapids, Michigan, USA

JESSE FORBES DOTY, MD
Assistant Professor and Director of Foot and Ankle Surgery, UT Erlanger Orthopaedics, The University of Tennessee College of Medicine, Chattanooga, Tennessee, USA

LELAND GOSSETT, MD
Resident, Spectrum Health-Michigan State University, Grand Rapids, Michigan, USA

WALLACE TAYLOR HARRIS, MD
Orthopaedic Surgery Resident, PGY-3, UT Erlanger Orthopaedics, The University of Tennessee College of Medicine, Chattanooga, Tennessee, USA

JIN SU KIM, MD, PhD
Department of Orthopedics, CM General Hospital, Seoul, Korea

WOO-CHUN LEE, MD
Seoul Foot and Ankle Center, Dubalo Orthopaedic Clinic, Seoul, Korea

LYNDON MASON, MBChB, MRCS, FRCS Tr&Orth
Consultant Orthopaedic Surgeon, Aintree University Hospital, Liverpool, Merseyside, United Kingdom; Honorary Clinical Senior Lecturer, Department of Musculoskeletal Biology, University of Liverpool, Liverpool, United Kingdom

ANDY MOLLOY, MBChB, MRCS, FRCS Tr&Orth
Consultant Orthopaedic Surgeon, Aintree University Hospital, Liverpool, Merseyside, United Kingdom; Honorary Clinical Senior Lecturer, Department of Musculoskeletal Biology, University of Liverpool, Liverpool, United Kingdom

RYUZO OKUDA, MD, PhD
Department of Orthopaedic Surgery, Shimizu Hospital, Kyoto, Japan

CRISTIAN ORTIZ, MD
Staff Member, Head of Foot and Ankle Unit, Orthopedic and Traumatology Department, Clinica Alemana, Associate Professor, Universidad del Desarrollo, Santiago, Chile

ANTHONY PERERA, MBChB, MRCS, MFSEM, PG Dip (Med Law), FRCS (Orth)
Consultant Orthopaedic Foot and Ankle Surgeon, Trauma and Orthopaedic Department, University Hospital of Wales, Cardiff, United Kingdom

ROBERT D. SANTROCK, MD
Associate Professor, Department of Orthopaedics, West Virginia University, Morgantown, West Virginia, USA

BRET SMITH, DO, MSc
Clinical Professor, Foot and Ankle Division, Moore Center for Orthopedics, Lexington, South Carolina, USA

NIALL A. SMYTH, MD
Orthopaedic Surgery Resident, Department of Orthopaedic Surgery, University of Miami, Miami, Florida, USA

ERIC SWANTON, MBChB, BA, BHB, FRACS (Orth)
Foot and Ankle Fellow, Aintree University Hospital, Liverpool, Merseyside, United Kingdom

EMILIO WAGNER, MD
Staff Member, Foot and Ankle Unit, Orthopedic and Traumatology Department, Clinica Alemana, Associate Professor, Universidad del Desarrollo, Santiago, Chile

PABLO WAGNER, MD
Staff Member, Foot and Ankle Unit, Orthopedic and Traumatology Department, Clinica Alemana, Associate Professor, Universidad del Desarrollo, Staff Member, Hospital Militar - Universidad de los Andes, Santiago, Chile

MATTHEW JAMES WELCK, MBChB, MSc, FRCS (Orth)
Consultant Orthopaedic Foot and Ankle Surgeon, Royal National Orthopaedic Hospital, London, United Kingdom

DANIEL M.G. WINSON, MBBS, MRCSEd
Trauma and Orthopaedic Department, University Hospital of Wales, Cardiff, United Kingdom

YOUNG YI, MD
Department of Orthopedic Surgery, Seoul Paik Hospital Inje University, Seoul, Korea

KI WON YOUNG, MD, PhD
Foot and Ankle Clinic, Department of Orthopedic Surgery, Eulji Medical Center, Eulji University School of Medicine, Seoul, Korea

Editorial Advisory Board

Contents

Niall A. Smyth and Amiethab A. Aiyer

Hallux valgus is a common pathology of the foot and ankle. Surgical correction of the condition has been described as early as 1836. Since then, numerous different surgical techniques have been documented in the literature. One of the explanations as to why there are so many different surgeries for hallux valgus is the variety of etiologies attributed to causing the condition. This article discusses the causes associated with hallux valgus and describes a few of the surgeries commonly used to treat the deformity.

Matthew James Welck and Naji Al-Khudairi

This article describes the pathogenesis of hallux valgus (HV) and the traditional ways to image the deformities. It also discusses up-to-date advances and research in the field of imaging in HV, including weight-bearing computed tomography scanning, MRI, ultrasound scanning, and intraoperative imaging.

Young Yi and Woo-Chun Lee

Hallux valgus is a slowly progressing complex three-dimensional biomechanical process. Therefore, precise understanding of the three-dimensional deformity is essential for satisfactory clinical result. Uniplanar correction on anteroposterior view of foot would be insufficient, and rotation on the frontal plane as well as sagittal alignment should also be well corrected. This article reviews the three-dimensional components of bony displacement in different surgical methods for hallux valgus correction.

Pablo Wagner and Emilio Wagner

Rotational deformity in hallux valgus is a recognized component and a demonstrated recurrence factor in patients who have undergone surgery. More than 20 years ago, publications started reporting metatarsal pronation as part of the hallux valgus pathology. Identifying metatarsal pronation should be part of the preoperative angular measurements. The proximal metatarsal rotational osteotomy and Lapidus fusion are some of the few techniques that reliably correct metatarsal pronation. They have good results, with more nonunions reported for the Lapidus. The authors present

correction. The proximal oblique sliding closing wedge osteotomy follows the CORA concept and permits preoperative planning. Future directions must include the correction of the pronation deformity of the metatarsal.

Proximal Supination Osteotomy of the First Metatarsal for Hallux Valgus   257

Ryuzo Okuda

Postoperative recurrence of hallux valgus is a relatively common complication and is associated with unsatisfactory surgical outcomes. Risk factors for postoperative recurrence include a round lateral edge of the first metatarsal head (a positive round sign) and incomplete reduction of the sesamoids. These risk factors may relate to residual pronation of the first metatarsal following surgery. A novel technique of a proximal supination osteotomy, in which varus and pronation of the first metatarsal can be corrected simultaneously, can achieve significant correction in moderate or severe hallux valgus deformity and a low rate of hallux valgus recurrence.

Hallux Valgus Deformity and Treatment: A Three-Dimensional Approach   271

Jesse Forbes Doty and Wallace Taylor Harris

The cause and effect between hallux valgus and first ray hypermobility continues to be debated. Understanding the anatomic and radiographic examination of the first metatarsocuneiform (MTC) joint is critical to choosing an appropriate treatment algorithm for the surgical management of hallux valgus deformity. Some studies suggest that hypermobility can be corrected without fusing the first MTC joint. Some think hypermobility arises secondarily from malalignment of the soft tissue constraints as the hallux valgus deformity progresses. Others think hypermobility is a primary cause of the hallux valgus deformity and have reported good results with surgical correction, including a first tarsometatarsal arthrodesis.

Hallux Valgus Deformity and Treatment: A Three-Dimensional Approach: Modified Technique for Lapidus Procedure   281

Robert D. Santrock and Bret Smith

In a hallux valgus deformity, the problem is deviation of the hallux at the metatarsophalangeal joint and of the first metatarsal at the tarsometatarsal joint. Although anteroposterior radiograph findings have been prioritized, deviation in the other planes can substantially change visible cues. The modified technique for Lapidus procedure uses all 3 planes to evaluate and correct the deformity, making radiographic measurements less useful. Using a triplane framework and focusing on the apex of the deformity, all bunions become the same. Modified technique for Lapidus procedure can be performed regardless of the degree of deformity, always includes triplane correction, and deformity size becomes irrelevant.

Hallux Valgus/Medial Column Instability and Their Relationship with Posterior Tibial Tendon Dysfunction   297

Steven Blackwood and Leland Gossett

Historically, bunions have focused on the coronal plane; however, there is tension and compression failure in the sagittal plane of the midfoot during arch collapse. Correction of all 3 planes of deformity, coronal, sagittal, and rotational, can be achieved in several ways. Taking a big picture of global foot mechanics by recognizing the common types of conditions associated with arch collapse, including hallux valgus deformities, can serve as a useful roadmap for navigating more complicated deformities where hallux valgus exists.

FOOT AND ANKLE CLINICS

THE CLINICS ARE NOW AVAILABLE ONLINE!
Access your subscription at:
www.theclinics.com

Preface

Hallux Valgus: A Three-Dimensional Approach

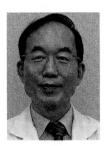

Woo-Chun Lee, MD
Editor

Hallux valgus is a common deformity that often requires surgical correction. Therefore, every foot and ankle surgeon is familiar with several procedures for hallux valgus deformity. However, there are many recurrences and complications after hallux valgus surgery.

The title of this issue, "Hallux Valgus: A Three-Dimensional Approach," conveys the contents of this issue of *Foot and Ankle Clinics of North America*. This issue was written to review the current approaches to the hallux valgus correction, the three-dimensional change of the first metatarsal, and the first metatarsocuneiform joint in hallux valgus. Coronal plane deformity is then discussed as the possible cause of recurrences of hallux valgus surgery, and various techniques of three-dimensional correction are introduced as an answer to the question of why the hallux valgus deformity recurs.

Gross deformity and plain radiographs show only the transverse plane deformity, and correction in the transverse plane is the primary object of hallux valgus surgery, which explains why current methods of two-dimensional correction are so popular.

Contrary to the traditional concept of hallux valgus as a two-dimensional deformity, a concept that the hallux valgus is a three-dimensional deformity was developed by several authors a long time ago; however, practical methods to take care of those three-dimensional deformities have only recently drawn the interest of many surgeons after experiencing unsuccessful results.

Better understanding of the three-dimensional approach was the result of several recent articles, and several different surgical techniques have been developed to fix the three-dimensional deformity based on those reports. Supination at the osteotomy site or at the first tarsometatarsal joint constitutes the principal method of correcting the three-dimensional deformity, and several techniques of different authors are introduced in this issue.

Foot Ankle Clin N Am 23 (2018) xiii–xiv
https://doi.org/10.1016/j.fcl.2018.03.001
1083-7515/18/© 2018 Published by Elsevier Inc.

    I believe this issue is helpful in developing a more reasonable approach to the hallux valgus by providing a deeper understanding of three-dimensional geometry and also by learning techniques for the correction of the three-dimensional deformity.

Woo-Chun Lee, MD
Seoul Foot and Ankle Center
Dubalo Orthopaedic Clinic
Dongjak-Daero 212
Seocho-Gu, Seoul 06554, Korea

E-mail address:
leewoochun@gmail.com

Introduction: Why Are There so Many Different Surgeries for Hallux Valgus?

Niall A. Smyth, MD, Amiethab A. Aiyer, MD*

KEYWORDS

• Hallux valgus • Bunion • Etiology • Chevron • Lapidus • Scarf

KEY POINTS

- More than 100 different surgical procedures have been described for the treatment of hallux valgus.
- Multiple etiologic factors have been linked to the development of hallux valgus, potentially explaining the multitude of surgical procedures available to correct the deformity.
- Despite the variety of surgical options for treating hallux valgus, there is no gold standard.

INTRODUCTION

An important pathology of the foot, namely, hallux valgus (HV), is ever present in a foot and ankle surgeon's practice and widely discussed in the literature. Invariably common, the prevalence of HV in the general public has been reported to potentially be between 23.0% and 35.7%.[1–3] In 1994, it was estimated that approximately 209,000 HV surgeries were performed annually in the United States.[4] The number of patients undergoing deformity correction is surely much higher currently. Despite the widespread presence of the pathology, there is no shortage of surgical options to address HV.

ETIOLOGY
Extrinsic Causes

One of the possible reasons for the diversity of surgical options for HV is the spectrum of etiologies of the deformity. Footwear was one of the early explanations given for the development of HV. Thought to be an extrinsic cause as early as 1909, high heels and

The authors have nothing to disclose.
Department of Orthopaedic Surgery, University of Miami, 1611 Northwest 12th Avenue, Miami, FL 33136, USA
* Corresponding author.
E-mail address: tabsaiyer@gmail.com

narrow toe-box shoes are frequently associated with HV.[5] Although increasing heel height increases forefoot loading,[6] there is not complete penetrance of HV in women who wear high heels. It is possible, however, that abnormal forefoot loading caused by high heels may exacerbate the deformity.[7] In addition, there is no link between footwear and the development of juvenile HV.[8]

Intrinsic Causes

Multiple intrinsic factors have been evaluated as causes of HV. These include a long first metatarsal, the shape of the metatarsal head, and soft tissue imbalances across the hallux metatarsophalangeal (MP) joint. A long first metatarsal has been thought to be a risk factor for development of HV. In a study assessing patients with HV, it was found that 80% had a zero-plus first metatarsal (first metatarsal greater or equal in length when compared with the second metatarsal). This finding is in contrast to control subjects, of whom 80% had a shorter first metatarsal.[9] Another anatomic variant linked with HV is a round first metatarsal head. Although the flattened or square-shaped head is considered more stable,[10,11] a rounded head has been reported to be unstable and may be at higher risk for HV recurrence after surgical intervention.[12] It is important to consider that there is no accurate method of describing the metatarsal head and its appearance may change depending on metatarsal supination and pronation. Therefore, it is not clear as to whether anatomic variants of the first metatarsal directly cause HV.

The static stabilizers of the first MP joint are often compromised in order for the deformity to develop. The collateral ligament, medial sesamoid ligament, and joint capsule make up the medial restraints. In the presence of HV, these structures are mechanically attenuated and have abnormal collagen organization at the histologic level.[13] However, it is more likely that pathology of these structures is due to HV, rather than a cause.[14] The dynamic stabilizers of the first MP also play a role and show muscle imbalance in the presence of deformity. These stabilizers include the adductor hallucis and abductor hallucis, with the latter causing great toe plantarflexion and abduction.[15] With regard to the extensor and flexor hallucis longus, as the deformity progresses, the moment arm of the extensor hallucis longus and flexor hallucis longus migrates laterally. This augments the deforming force of the muscle to pull the toe into valgus.[16,17]

Other kinematic factors of the foot have been linked with HV. As an example, hypermobility of the first ray in the sagittal plane and its role in HV is a source of significant discussion in the orthopedic literature. Hypermobility of the first ray may lead to elevation of the first metatarsal, which results in increased pronation, increased medial load on the MP joint, and valgus stress on the hallux.[18] This finding has led some authors to argue that there is increased recurrence of HV if the tarsometatarsal joint has not been fused.[19] Others have demonstrated that sagittal plane hypermobility improves with osteotomies alone.[20] It is important to also consider hypermobility in the coronal plane, which can lead to medial deviation of the metatarsal and subsequent HV. This factor may potentially be more important than sagittal plane mobility, because the latter has not been proven to be a definitive cause.[21] Another kinematic variant implicated in HV is a tight Achilles tendon, causing increased forefoot loading.[22–24] Although there have been reports of an association between HV and decreased ankle dorsiflexion,[10,25] other authors have not discovered the same relationship.[26]

Last, pes planus has been associated with HV deformity with multiple potential biomechanical reasons. The deformity causes an elevation of the first ray and, therefore, a functional long first metatarsal.[27] In addition, the peroneus longus is less able to stabilize the first metatarsal and collapse of the midfoot can lead to hypermobility of the first ray.[28,29] As the pes planus deformity worsens, there is increased pronation on the first ray leading to loading of the plantar medial border of the hallux, placing undue strain over the stabilizers of the MP joint.[30] Despite the seemingly logical link between the 2 deformities, Coughlin and Jones[10] found no association between measures of HV and pes planus. Furthermore, if pes planus caused HV owing to the factors as described, it would be reasonable to expect a higher risk of recurrence after surgical correction. This outcome, however, has not been found to be true.[22,31,32]

Regardless of the cause of HV, the deformity progresses in a relatively predictable manner. The metatarsal head migrates medially, uncovering the sesamoid complex. The abductor hallucis, which provides medial sided dynamic stability, falls plantarward. The proximal phalanx drifts into a valgus deformity as it remains attached to the adductor hallucis and sesamoids. The deforming force of the adductor hallucis is amplified by the abductor hallucis. The metatarsal head pronates as it falls off the sesamoids and, as stated, the extensor hallucis longus and flexor hallucis longus tendons bowstring laterally. The thin and structurally weaker, dorsomedial MP capsule provides poor medial static stability. Last, the bursa over the joint thickens over time with the pressure of footwear on the medial eminence[14] (**Fig. 1**).

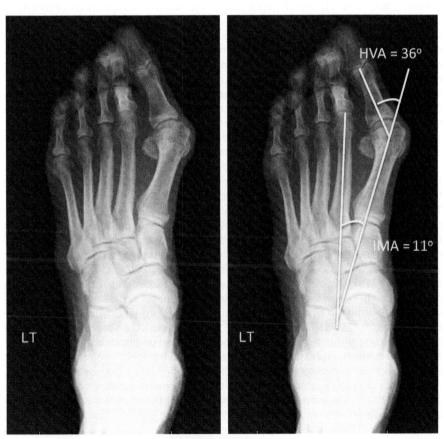

Fig. 1. Hallux valgus of the left foot with illustration of the hallux valgus angle (HVA) and intermetatarsal angle (IMA).

Extrinsic factors (eg, shoewear), anatomic variants (eg, metatarsal length and head shape), and kinematic changes (eg, hypermobility) have all been implicated in the development of HV with conflicting findings in the literature. The complexity regarding the etiology of HV has led to an enormous variety of surgical procedures to address the deformity. As will be discussed, some surgical options attempt to address the first metatarsal anatomy, whereas others try to correct for deficient static stabilizers or kinematic variants.

SURGICAL OPTIONS

Easley and Trnka[33] reported that more than 100 different operative procedures have been described to treat HV. Starting with the most basic surgical correction, a procedure consisting of resecting the medial eminence and imbrication of the MP joint capsule has been described as a bunionectomy. However, given the low rate of patient satisfaction and high risk of recurrence,[34] the procedure is not commonly used in modern practice. The other soft tissue procedure that has been used in isolation is the modified McBride procedure. This consists of an MP joint lateral capsulotomy, adductor hallucis release, division of the ligament between the lateral capsule and fibular sesamoid, and imbrication of the medial capsule.[33,35] The principle of this technique is to only address the soft tissue causes of HV with correction of the muscle imbalances and imbrication of the medial stabilizers. Although there have been reports of acceptable patient satisfaction rates,[36] as the understanding of the etiology of HV has evolved, this soft tissue procedure is now commonly combined with other osseous corrective techniques. This is due to improved understanding of the etiologies causing HV and the realization that addressing only the soft tissue pathology is unlikely to be sufficient. Variances of an isolated lateral soft tissue release have also been described, with techniques including a dorsal, intermetatarsal webspace, and an intraarticular approach.[37] Addressing both the soft tissue and osseous components of the deformity are critical to restore static and dynamic balance across the hallux MP joint. These other techniques are diverse and frequently subdivided into distal and proximal procedures.

One of the most commonly used distal osteotomies is the chevron osteotomy, with the distal fragment shifted laterally (**Fig. 2**).[38] Multiple studies have confirmed that this technique achieves acceptable outcomes with significant patient satisfaction.[39–42] The combination of the chevron osteotomy with a soft tissue procedure (eg, adductor release) highlights the importance of balancing all facets of deforming forces across the hallux MP joint and addressing the various etiologies. Resch and colleagues[43] published a study reporting the results comparing the chevron with a lateral release, versus a chevron in isolation. The authors reported that although the radiographic correction was significantly improved in the combined procedure, patient satisfaction did not differ between the groups. An additional surgical option with regard to the chevron osteotomy is whether to perform the procedure in a minimally invasive or open fashion.[44,45] Brogan and colleagues[46] recently reported on the results of a cohort study assessing the minimally invasive technique versus the traditional open technique. The authors report that the clinical and radiographic postoperative scores were significantly improved in both groups with no difference between the 2 groups. Another consideration is the variety of surgical fixation options that have been described.[39,41,47] Therefore, within just the realm of the chevron osteotomy, there are a multitude of options to address HV. With regard to complications of the chevron, osteonecrosis of the metatarsal head is of concern, particularly with penetration of the dorsolateral branches of the first dorsal metatarsal artery.[37,48] The osteotomy disrupts the vascular supply to the metatarsal head, which may potentially be further damaged

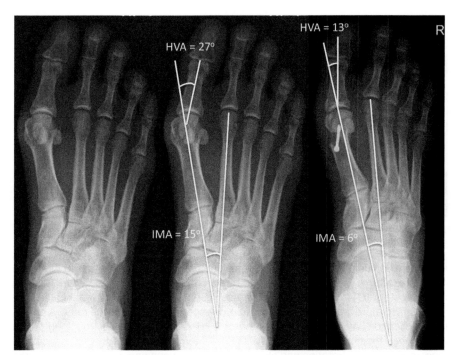

Fig. 2. Anteroposterior radiographs of preoperative and postoperative right foot after chevron osteotomy with illustration of the hallux valgus angle (HVA) and intermetatarsal angle (IMA).

if the procedure is combined with a soft tissue release.[49] However, this procedure has not been shown to be associated with an increased risk of avascular necrosis.[49,50]

Traditionally, patients exhibiting a more severe deformity may be treated with proximal first metatarsal osteotomies. Multiple surgical techniques exist for proximal osteotomies, including performing a proximal chevron. This procedure combines the corrective translation technique of the distal chevron with the creation of an opening wedge.[51,52] The crescentic osteotomy has also been described as an option for proximal correction. The technique requires a specialized crescentic saw blade and has been noted to be technically challenging.[53] The crescentic osteotomy has been shown to provide successful results, although there are reports that it has a relatively high rate of dorsiflexion malunion.[54,55] Of note, there are fewer publications in the recent literature regarding this technique, potentially indicating decreased popularity. The Ludloff osteotomy is another proximal procedure that has been described consisting of an oblique osteotomy. The technique has been shown to result in an acceptable improvement of the deformity and clinical scores.[56,57] A concern regarding the Ludloff technique is shortening of the metatarsal, with Choi and colleagues[57] demonstrating an average decrease in length of 2.6 mm. This effect may be beneficial if the goal of the surgery is to also address an anatomic variant of a long first metatarsal that may be potentially contributing to the HV deformity. However, it may not be appropriate in a patient with a short first ray or metatarsalgia.

An additional procedure that has gained popularity, particularly outside the United States is the scarf osteotomy. The procedure is a midshaft Z-shaped osteotomy with a dorsal distal limb and plantar proximal limb (**Fig. 3**).[58] Arguments in favor of the scarf osteotomy are that it provides potentially greater correction than other

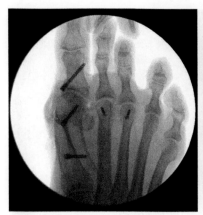
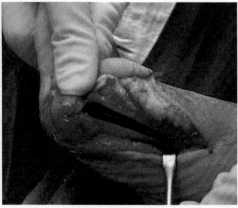

Fig. 3. Intraoperative and fluoroscopic image showing the Scarf osteotomy.

techniques, including correction of the distal metatarsal articular angle, and that it is a stable osteotomy. However, in a randomized control comparing the scarf with the chevron osteotomy, Jeuken and colleagues[59] concluded that both techniques provided similar improvements in clinical outcomes scores and recurrence rates. A potential complication unique to the scarf osteotomy is the phenomenon of troughing, which occurs when the hard cortical edges of the osteotomy wedge into the soft cancellous bone, resulting in malrotation and elevation. Troughing can occur when the dorsal and plantar limbs are larger than 2 to 3 mm (subsequently cutting into cancellous bone), completing the osteotomy in osteoporotic or osteopenic bone, or overcompression with screw fixation.[60] A rotational technique has been proposed as a solution to decrease this complication.[61] Again, as is the trend with most of the different surgical procedures used to treat HV, there are instances of complications secondary to the technique[60]; however the vast majority of the reports indicate successful results. Bock and colleagues[62] published the results of a large case series at a mean follow-up of more than 10 years. The authors noted that there was a significant mean improvement in clinical outcome scores, without evidence of troughing. However, the authors noted a recurrence rate of 30% at final follow-up.

Other important surgical tools for HV correction are based on the principle of stabilizing the first tarsometatarsal joint. One option is the modified Lapidus procedure, which is an arthrodesis of this articulation (**Fig. 4**).[63] This is in contrast to the original description of the procedure, which consists of an arthrodesis of the first tarsometatarsal joint, augmented by an intermetatarsal joint arthrodesis to address coronal plane instability.[64] Indications for this procedure include a severe deformity and arthritis of the tarsometatarsal joint. In addition, it is used when the surgeon believes that the greatest contributing etiology to the HV deformity is hypermobility of the first ray.[63] Again, there are a variety of fixation techniques that have been described with the Lapidus procedure, with interfragmentary screw and locking plate versus interfragmentary screw fixation alone being the most common.[65] Both techniques have shown good clinical outcomes.[66–68] There are 2 principle concerns regarding the Lapidus procedure. The first is a potential nonunion, with the literature indicating a rate of approximately 2% to 10%.[63,69–71] The second concern is shortening and dorsiflexion of the first ray, leading to transfer metatarsalgia.[72,73]

A separate procedure that can be used to treat HV is a hallux MP arthrodesis (**Fig. 5**). This procedure is usually considered in patients with severe deformity, in the presence

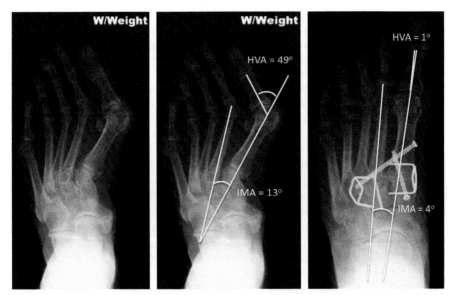

Fig. 4. Anteroposterior radiographs of preoperative and postoperative left foot after first tarsometatarsal joint arthrodesis with supplemental arthrodesis of second and third tarsometatarsal joints. Illustration of the hallux valgus angle (HVA) and intermetatarsal angle (IMA).

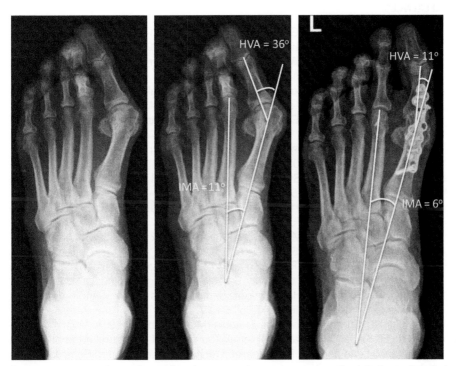

Fig. 5. Anteroposterior radiographs of preoperative and postoperative left foot after first metatarsophalangeal joint arthrodesis with illustration of the hallux valgus angle (HVA) and intermetatarsal angle (IMA).

of arthritis, and for those suffering from a neuromuscular disorder.[33] Furthermore, the procedure potentially counters several etiologies implicated in the deformity, including a long first metatarsal, a round metatarsal head, and dynamic muscled imbalances. In addition, Coughlin and colleagues[74] have demonstrated that it may be used as an option for the revision of a previously failed HV surgery. This includes patients with a hypermobile first ray; the authors showed that there was no evidence of hypermobility after MP arthrodesis.[75] The surgery has been shown to result in successful outcomes, with evidence of correction of the intermetatarsal angle.[76] An issue with arthrodesis of the first MP joint is whether it should be combined with a proximal corrective osteotomy of the first metatarsal. This is due to conflicting evidence in the literature regarding adequate deformity correction with using a fusion in isolation.[77–79]

SUMMARY

There are a variety of operative options to address an HV deformity. The concept of correcting the deformity surgically has been around for over a century and half, with Trnka and colleagues[80] noting that the earliest surgery occurred in 1836. The diversity of the surgeries available is partially due to the multiple etiologic factors attributable to causing HV. Many of these surgeries are still in use today, and although the severity of the disease may affect the reasoning regarding choosing a certain procedure, it is ultimately up to the surgeon's preference. Although multiple comparison studies have been published assessing the outcomes of different techniques,[57,81–85] there is no consensus in the literature as to which is the gold standard for treating HV.

REFERENCES

1. Benvenuti F, Ferrucci L, Guralnik JM, et al. Foot pain and disability in older persons: an epidemiologic survey. J Am Geriatr Soc 1995;43(5):479–84.
2. Elton PJ, Sanderson SP. A chiropodial survey of elderly persons over 65 years in the community. Public Health 1986;100(4):219–22.
3. Nix S, Smith M, Vicenzino B. Prevalence of hallux valgus in the general population: a systematic review and meta-analysis. J Foot Ankle Res 2010;3:21.
4. Coughlin MJ, Thompson FM. The high price of high-fashion footwear. Instr Course Lect 1995;44:371–7.
5. Porter JL. Why operations for bunion fail with a description of one that does not. Surg Gynecol Obstet 1909;8:89.
6. Corrigan JP, Moore DP, Stephens MM. Effect of heel height on forefoot loading. Foot Ankle 1993;14:148–52.
7. Hughes J, Clark P, Jagoe RR, et al. The pattern of pressure distribution under the weightbearing forefoot. Foot 1991;1:117–24.
8. Coughlin MJ. Roger A. Mann Award. Juvenile hallux valgus: etiology and treatment. Foot Ankle Int 1995;16:682–97.
9. Mancuso JE, Abramow SP, Landsman MJ, et al. The zeroplus first metatarsal and its relationship to bunion deformity. J Foot Ankle Surg 2003;42:319–26.
10. Coughlin MJ, Jones CP. Hallux valgus: demographics, etiology, and radiographic assessment. Foot Ankle Int 2007;28:759–77.
11. DuVries HL. Surgery of the foot. St Louis (MO): Mosby; 1959.
12. Okuda R, Kinoshita M, Yasuda T, et al. The shape of the lateral edge of the first metatarsal head as a risk factor for recurrence of hallux valgus. J Bone Joint Surg Am 2007;89:2163–72.
13. Uchiyama E, Kitaoka HB, Luo ZP, et al. Pathomechanics of hallux valgus: biomechanical and immunohistochemical study. Foot Ankle Int 2005;26:732–8.

14. Perera AM, Mason L, Stephens MM. The pathogenesis of hallux valgus. J Bone Joint Surg Am 2011;93(17):1650–61.
15. Arinci Incel N, Gencx H, Erdem HR, et al. Muscle imbalance in hallux valgus: an electromyographic study. Am J Phys Med Rehabil 2003;82:345–9.
16. Lamur KS, Huson A, Snijders CJ, et al. Geometric data of hallux valgus feet. Foot Ankle Int 1996;17:548–54.
17. Saltzman CL, Aper RL, Brown TD. Anatomic determinants of first metatarsophalangeal flexion moments in hallux valgus. Clin Orthop Relat Res 1997;339:261–9.
18. Dananberg HJ. Functional hallux limitus and its relationship to gait efficiency. J Am Podiatr Med Assoc 1986;76:648–52.
19. McNerney JE, Johnston WB. Generalized ligamentous laxity, hallux abducto valgus and the first metatarsocuneiform joint. J Am Podiatry Assoc 1979;69:69–82.
20. Coughlin MJ, Jones CP. Hallux valgus and first ray mobility. A prospective study. J Bone Joint Surg Am 2007;89:1887–98.
21. Doty JF, Coughlin MJ. Hallux valgus and hypermobility of the first ray: facts and fiction. Int Orthop 2013;37(9):1655–60.
22. Mann RA, Coughlin MJ. Hallux valgus—etiology, anatomy, treatment and surgical considerations. Clin Orthop Relat Res 1981;157:31–41.
23. Hansen ST Jr. Hallux valgus surgery. Morton and Lapidus were right! Clin Podiatr Med Surg 1996;13:347–54.
24. Ward ED, Phillips RD, Patterson PE, et al. 1998 William J. Stickel Gold Award. The effects of extrinsic muscle forces on the forefoot-to-rearfoot loading relationship in vitro. Tibia and Achilles tendon. J Am Podiatr Med Assoc 1998;88:471–82.
25. Di Giovanni CW, Kuo R, Tejwani N, et al. Isolated gastrocnemius tightness. J Bone Joint Surg Am 2000;84:962–70.
26. Veri JP, Pirani SP, Claridge R. Crescentic proximal metatarsal osteotomy for moderate to severe hallux valgus: a mean 12.2 year follow-up study. Foot Ankle Int 2001;22:817–22.
27. Phillips RD, Phillips RL. Quantitative analysis of the locking position of the midtarsal joint. J Am Podiatry Assoc 1983;73:518–22.
28. Donatelli RA. Normal biomechanics of the foot and ankle. J Orthop Sports Phys Ther 1985;7:91–5.
29. Tiberio D. Pathomechanics of structural foot deformities. Phys Ther 1988;68:1840–9.
30. Phillips D. Biomechanics in hallux valgus and forefoot surgery. In: Hetherington VJ, editor. Hallux valgus and forefoot surgery. New York: Churchill and Livingstone; 2000. p. 44.
31. Canale PB, Aronsson DD, Lamont RL, et al. The Mitchell procedure for the treatment of adolescent hallux valgus. A long-term study. J Bone Joint Surg Am 1993;75:1610–8.
32. Kilmartin TE, Wallace WA. The significance of pes planus in juvenile hallux valgus. Foot Ankle 1992;13:53–6.
33. Easley ME, Trnka HJ. Current concepts review: hallux valgus part II: operative treatment. Foot Ankle Int 2007;28(6):748–58.
34. Kitaoka HB, Franco MG, Weaver AL, et al. Simple bunionectomy with medial capsulorrhaphy. Foot Ankle 1991;12:86–91.
35. Pfeffinger LL. The modified McBride procedure. Orthopedics 1990;13:979–84.
36. Mann RA, Pfeffinger L. Hallux valgus repair. DuVries modified McBride procedure. Clin Orthop 1991;272:213–8.

37. Jones KJ, Feiwell LA, Freedman EL, et al. The effect of chevron osteotomy with lateral capsular release on the blood supply to the first metatarsal head. J Bone Joint Surg Am 1995;77(2):197–204.

38. Austin DW, Leventen EO. A new osteotomy for hallux valgus: a horizontally directed "V" displacement osteotomy of the metatarsal head for hallux valgus and primus varus. Clin Orthop 1981;157:25–30.

39. Crosby LA, Bozarth GR. Fixation comparison for chevron osteotomies. Foot Ankle Int 1998;19:41–3.

40. Deorio JK, Ware AW. Single absorbable polydioxanone pin fixation for distal chevron bunion osteotomies. Foot Ankle Int 2001;22:832–5.

41. Gill LH, Martin DF, Coumas JM, et al. Fixation with bioabsorbable pins in chevron bunionectomy. J Bone Joint Surg 1997;79-A:1510–8.

42. Mann RA, Donatto KC. The chevron osteotomy: a clinical and radiographic analysis. Foot Ankle Int 1997;18:255–61.

43. Resch S, Stenstrom A, Reynisson K, et al. Chevron osteotomy for hallux valgus not improved by additional adductor tenotomy. A prospective, randomized study of 84 patients. Acta Orthop Scand 1994;65:541–4.

44. Lam P, Lee M, Xing J, et al. Percutaneous surgery for mild to moderate hallux valgus. Foot Ankle Clin 2016;21(3):459–77.

45. Vernois J, Redfern DJ. Percutaneous surgery for severe hallux valgus. Foot Ankle Clin 2016;21(3):479–93.

46. Brogan K, Lindisfarne E, Akehurst H, et al. Minimally invasive and open distal chevron osteotomy for mild to moderate hallux valgus. Foot Ankle Int 2016; 37(11):1197–204.

47. Plaass C, Ettinger S, Sonnow L, et al. Early results using a biodegradable magnesium screw for modified chevron osteotomies. J Orthop Res 2016;34(12): 2207–14.

48. Meier PJ, Kenzora JE. The risks and benefits of distal first metatarsal osteotomies. Foot Ankle 1985;6:7–17.

49. Kuhn MA, Lippert FG 3rd, Phipps MJ, et al. Blood flow to the metatarsal head after chevron bunionectomy. Foot Ankle Int 2005;26:526–9.

50. Resch S, Stenstrom A, Gustafson T. Circulatory disturbance of the first metatarsal head after chevron osteotomy as shown by bone scintigraphy. Foot Ankle 1992; 13:137–42.

51. Sammarco GJ, Conti SF. Proximal chevron metatarsal osteotomy: single incision technique. Foot Ankle 1993;14:44–7.

52. Sammarco GJ, Russo-Alesi FG. Bunion correction using proximal chevron osteotomy: a single-incision technique. Foot Ankle Int 1998;19:430–7.

53. Wester JU, Hamborg-Petersen E, Herold N, et al. Open wedge metatarsal osteotomy versus crescentic osteotomy to correct severe hallux valgus deformity – A prospective comparative study. Foot Ankle Surg 2016;22(1):26–31.

54. Markbreiter LA, Thompson FM. Proximal metatarsal osteotomy in hallux valgus correction: a comparison of crescentic and chevron procedures. Foot Ankle Int 1997;18:71–6.

55. Zettl R, Trnka HJ, Easley M, et al. Moderate to severe hallux valgus deformity: correction with proximal crescentic osteotomy and distal soft-tissue release. Arch Orthop Trauma Surg 2000;120:397–402.

56. Chiodo CP, Schon LC, Myerson MS. Clinical results with the Ludloff osteotomy for correction of adult hallux valgus. Foot Ankle Int 2004;25:532–6.

57. Choi WJ, Yoon HK, Yoon HS, et al. Comparison of the proximal chevron and Ludloff osteotomies for the correction of hallux valgus. Foot Ankle Int 2009;30: 1154–60.
58. Barouk LS. Scarf osteotomy for hallux valgus correction. Local anatomy, surgical technique, and combination with other forefoot procedures. Foot Ankle Clin 2000; 5:525–58.
59. Jeuken RM, Schotanus MG, Kort NP, et al. Long-term follow-up of a randomized controlled trial comparing scarf to chevron osteotomy in hallux valgus correction. Foot Ankle Int 2016;37(7):687–95.
60. Coetzee JC. Scarf osteotomy for hallux valgus repair: the dark side. Foot Ankle Int 2003;24:29–33.
61. Murawski CD, Egan CJ, Kennedy JG. A rotational scarf osteotomy decreases troughing when treating hallux valgus. Clin Orthop Relat Res 2011;469(3): 847–53.
62. Bock P, Kluger R, Kristen KH, et al. The scarf osteotomy with minimally invasive lateral release for treatment of hallux valgus deformity: intermediate and long-term results. J Bone Joint Surg Am 2015;97(15):1238–45.
63. Schmid T, Krause F. The modified Lapidus fusion. Foot Ankle Clin 2014;19(2): 223–33.
64. Lapidus PW. Operative correction of the metatarsus varus primus in hallux valgus. Surg Gynecol Obstet 1934;58:16.
65. Harrison WD, Walker CR. Controversies and trends in United Kingdom Bunion Surgery. Foot Ankle Clin 2016;21(2):207–17.
66. Cottom JM, Vora AM. Fixation of Lapidus arthrodesis with plantar interfragmentary screw and medial locking plate: a report of 88 cases. J Foot Ankle Surg 2013;52(4):465–9.
67. Klos K, Gueorguiev B, Mückley T, et al. Stability of medial locking plate and compression screw versus two crossed screws for Lapidus arthrodesis. Foot Ankle Int 2010;31(2):158–63.
68. Mani SB, Lloyd EW, MacMahon A, et al. Modified Lapidus procedure with joint compression, meticulous surface preparation, and strain-relieved bone graft yields low nonunion rate. HSS J 2015;11(3):243–8.
69. Sangeorzan BJ, Hansen ST Jr. Modified Lapidus procedure for hallux valgus. Foot Ankle 1989;9:262–6.
70. Myerson M, Allon S, McGarvey W. Metatarsocuneiform arthrodesis for management of hallux valgus and metatarsus primus varus. Foot Ankle 1992;13:107–15.
71. Patel S, Ford LA, Etcheverry J, et al. Modified Lapidus arthrodesis: rate of nonunion in 227 cases. J Foot Ankle Surg 2004;43:37–42.
72. Coetzee JC, Resig SG, Kuskowski M, et al. The Lapidus procedure as salvage after failed surgical treatment of hallux valgus: a prospective cohort study. J Bone Joint Surg Am 2003;85A:60–5.
73. Coetzee JC, Wickum D. The Lapidus procedure: a prospective cohort outcome study. Foot Ankle Int 2004;25:526–31.
74. Coughlin MJ, Grebing BR, Jones CP. Arthrodesis of the first metatarsophalangeal joint for idiopathic hallux valgus: intermediate results. Foot Ankle Int 2005;26(10): 783–92.
75. Grimes JS, Coughlin MJ. First metatarsophalangeal joint arthrodesis as a treatment for failed hallux valgus surgery. Foot Ankle Int 2006;27(11):887–93.
76. McKean RM, Bergin PF, Watson G, et al. Radiographic evaluation of intermetatarsal angle correction following first MTP joint arthrodesis for severe hallux valgus. Foot Ankle Int 2016;37(11):1183–6.

77. Rippstein PF, Park YU, Naal FD. Combination of first metatarsophalangeal joint arthrodesis and proximal correction for severe hallux valgus deformity. Foot Ankle Int 2012;33(5):400–5.

78. Dayton P. Letter regarding: radiographic evaluation of intermetarsal angle correction following first MTP joint arthrodesis for severe hallux valgus. Foot Ankle Int 2016;37(11):1187.

79. Bergin PF, McKean RM, Watson G, et al. Response to "letter regarding: radiographic evaluation of intermetarsal angle correction following first MTP joint arthrodesis for severe hallux valgus". Foot Ankle Int 2016;37(11):1188.

80. Trnka HJ, Krenn S, Schuh R. Minimally invasive hallux valgus surgery: a critical review of the evidence. Int Orthop 2013;37(9):1731–5.

81. Uygur E, Özkan NK, Akan K, et al. A comparison of chevron and Lindgren-Turan osteotomy techniques in hallux valgus surgery: a prospective randomized controlled study. Acta Orthop Traumatol Turc 2016;50(3):255–61.

82. Scharer BM, DeVries JG. Comparison of chevron and distal oblique osteotomy for bunion correction. J Foot Ankle Surg 2016;55(4):738–42.

83. Lee KB, Cho NY, Park HW, et al. A comparison of proximal and distal chevron osteotomy, both with lateral soft-tissue release, for moderate to severe hallux valgus in patients undergoing simultaneous bilateral correction: a prospective randomised controlled trial. Bone Joint J 2015;97-B(2):202–7.

84. Park YB, Lee KB, Kim SK, et al. Comparison of distal soft-tissue procedures combined with a distal chevron osteotomy for moderate to severe hallux valgus: first web-space versus transarticular approach. J Bone Joint Surg Am 2013; 95(21):e158.

85. Park CH, Jang JH, Lee SH, et al. A comparison of proximal and distal chevron osteotomy for the correction of moderate hallux valgus deformity. Bone Joint J 2013;95-B(5):649–56.

Imaging of Hallux Valgus
How to Approach the Deformity

Matthew James Welck, MBChB, MSc, FRCS (Orth)*, Naji Al-Khudairi, MBBS, BSc

KEYWORDS

- Imaging • Radiology • Hallux valgus • Weight-bearing computed tomography

KEY POINTS

- Hallux valgus is a multiplanar deformity with transverse, sagittal, and rotational aspects.
- Conventional imaging techniques help with quantifying and analyzing the deformity; however, they suffer from some reproducibility and accuracy issues.
- Newer techniques are allowing further research into the deformity, and may afford a better understanding and improve surgical planning and assessment of surgical outcomes.

INTRODUCTION

Hallux valgus was originally thought to be caused by an enlargement of the metatarsophalangeal joint of the great toe. The deformity was later described by Carl Hueter (1838–1882), a German surgeon, as a lateral deviation of the great toe at the metatarsophalangeal joint; the term hallux abducto-valgus was developed.[1]

ETIOLOGY AND PATHOANATOMY

Despite its frequency,[2,3] the etiology of HV remains somewhat disputed. The etiology is often usefully subdivided into intrinsic and extrinsic causes[4–8] as discussed in previous articles.

HV is a slowly progressive condition resulting from a series of biomechanical changes. There are several steps in the pathophysiology; however, they do not always occur sequentially.[1]

The medial supporting structures of the first metatarsophalangeal joint are the capsule, the medial metatarso-sesamoid ligaments, and medial collateral ligament. These stretch and fail, and this is felt to be an early and fundamental step. This then allows the metatarsal head to drift medially. As the metatarsal moves medially, the

Disclosure Statement: Dr F. Lintz is a consultant for Curvebeam, LLC. Dr M.J. Welck and Dr N. Al-Khudairi have nothing to disclose.
Royal National Orthopaedic Hospital, London, UK
* Corresponding author.
E-mail address: matthewwelck@doctors.org.uk

Foot Ankle Clin N Am 23 (2018) 183–192
https://doi.org/10.1016/j.fcl.2018.01.002
1083-7515/18/Crown Copyright © 2018 Published by Elsevier Inc. All rights reserved.

foot.theclinics.com

sesamoids remain tethered in position by the adductor hallucis tendon and the inter-metatarsal ligaments. The proximal phalanx is in turn tethered to the sesamoids; there-fore this moves into a valgus position. Furthermore, as the metatarsal slides over the sesamoids, the metatarsal crista erodes, and the lateral sesamoid can appear to sit in the intermetatarsal space. As the metatarsal head drops off the sesamoid apparatus, it pronates because of the muscle forces acting across it. This defunctions the abductor hallucis, which usually strongly resists valgus of the proximal phalanx. The extensor and flexor hallucis longus tendons now bowstring laterally, further increasing the valgus displacement and occasionally acting as dorsiflexors of the proximal phalanx. The bursa overlying the medial eminence thickens due to the pressure effect of foot-wear on a prominent medial eminence (**Figs. 1** and **2**).

An oblique or an unstable first tarsometatarsal joint may support this process.

TRADITIONAL IMAGING TECHNIQUES

Traditionally AP, lateral, and oblique view plain radiographs form the mainstay of im-aging in HV deformity. From these, various radiographic angles have been utilized to assess and quantify the radiographic deformity of HV (**Fig. 3**).[9]

Hallux Valgus Angle

Reference points are placed on the proximal and distal midmetaphyseal regions of the first metatarsal and proximal phalanx.[9] Axes are drawn through these reference points on the first metatarsal and proximal phalanx. The angle created by the intersection of these axes is the hallux valgus angle (HVA). A normal angle is less than 15°, mild deformity less than 20°, moderate deformity 20 to 40°, and severe deformity greater than 40°. There are many discrepancies over these boundaries in the literature.

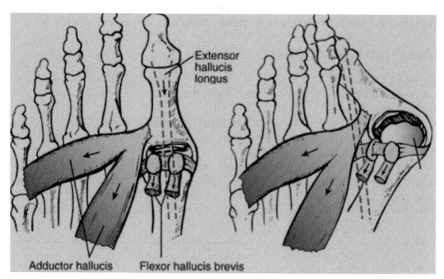

Fig. 1. This shows the metatarsal head moving into varus, and the sesamoids being tethered in place by the adductor hallucis tendon and the intermetatarsal ligament. It also demon-strates how the extensor hallucis tendon acts as a bowstring to perpetuate the deformity. (*From* Welck MJ, Singh D, Cullen N, et al. Evaluation of the 1st metatarso-sesamoid joint us-ing standing CT - the Stanmore classification. Foot Ankle Surg 2017;[pii:S1268-7731(17) 30059-0]; with permission.)

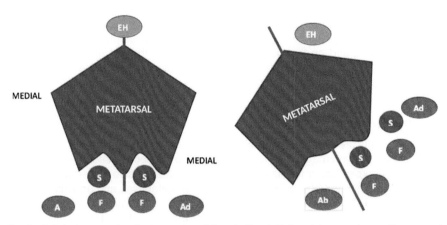

Fig. 2. Axial view at the first metatarsal head. The left hand image shows the normal, balanced situation. The right hand image shows pronation of the metatarsal head, with sesamoids (S), abductor (Ab), adductor (Ad), flexor hallucis brevis (F), and extensor hallucis (E) displacing and rotating relatively laterally. It also shows erosion of the crista underneath the metatarsal head.

Furthermore, where there is diaphyseal angulation, or after metatarsal osteotomy, an alternative is to use the center of the metatarsal head as a reference point.

1-2 Intermetatarsal Angle

Reference points are placed on the proximal and distal midmetaphyseal regions of the first and second metatarsals.[9] Axes are drawn through these reference points on the first and second metatarsals. The angle created by the intersection of these axes is the 1-2 IMA. Normal is less than 9°, mild deformity 9° to 11°, moderate deformity 12° to 16°, and severe deformity greater than 16°.

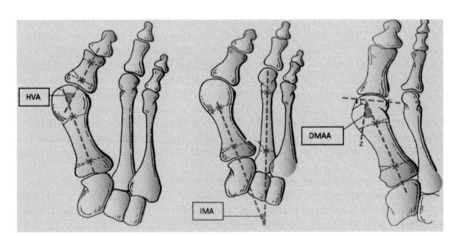

Fig. 3. Diagram showing the technique of measurement HVA, IMA, and distal metatarsal articular angle (DMAA). (*From* Welck MJ, Singh D, Cullen N, et al. Evaluation of the 1st metatarso-sesamoid joint using standing CT - the Stanmore classification. Foot Ankle Surg 2017;[pii:S1268-7731(17)30059-0]; with permission.)

Hallux Valgus Interphalangeal Angle

Reference points are placed on the proximal and distal midmetaphyseal regions of the proximal phalanx, and on the distal tip and midpoint of the articular surface of the distal phalanx.[9] Axes are drawn through these reference points on the proximal and distal phalanges. The angle created by the intersection of these axes is the hallux valgus interphalangeal (HVIP) angle.

Distal Metatarsal Articular Angle

Reference points are placed on the most medial and lateral aspect of the distal articular surface of the first metatarsal.[9] A line is drawn to connect these 2 points. Another line is drawn perpendicular to this line. Reference points are also placed on the proximal and distal midmetaphyseal regions of the first metatarsal, and an axis is drawn through the points. The angle subtended by the perpendicular line and first metatarsal longitudinal axes is the distal metatarsal articular angle (DMAA). Normal is less than 7°.

Metatarsophalangeal Joint Congruency

Reference points are placed on the most medial and lateral aspects of the articular surfaces of the first metatarsal head and base of the proximal phalanx.[9] The congruency of the metatarsophalangeal joint (MTPJ) is determined by assessing the relationship of the articular surfaces of the first metatarsal head with the base of the proximal phalanx. With a non-congruent HV deformity, the reference points on the base of proximal phalanx migrate laterally in relation to the points on the first metatarsal head. With a congruent MTPJ, the points remain aligned; there is no lateral shift of the proximal phalanx.

LIMITATIONS OF TRADITIONAL IMAGING TECHNIQUES

Given their widespread use in current clinical practice, studies have attempted to quantify the reliability of the aforementioned angular measurements. Coughlin and colleagues[10] investigated the intraobserver and inter-observer reliability and consistency of angular measurements in HV deformity. They evaluated the HVA, IMA, DMAA, and MTPJ congruency. Twenty-four orthopedic surgeons were recruited in the study. They found the IMA was measured within 5° or less in 96.7% of cases. The HVA was measured within 5° or less in 86.2% of cases. However, the DMAA was only measured to 5° or less in 58.9% of cases, and the range of MTPJ congruency varied from all 11 cases being identified to only 2 cases being identified. The authors concluded that although the study validates the reliability of IMA and HVA measurements, the reliability of DMAA and MTPJ congruency is questionable, largely because of difficulty in consistently identifying the most medial and lateral aspects of the articular surfaces.

Furthermore, as described, HV is a triplanar deformity comprised of a valgus deformity of the proximal phalanx, a pronation deformity of the first metatarsal, and a lateral displacement of the sesamoid apparatus. The standard imaging of HV deformity with two-dimensional (2D) plain radiographs provides limited information because of the rotational, three-dimensional nature of the deformity.

Modern advancements in clinical imaging have allowed the foot and ankle surgeon to utilize novel radiological techniques to better evaluate the pathogenesis and deformity of HV.

COMPUTED TOMOGRAPHY, SIMULATED WEIGHT-BEARING COMPUTED TOMOGRAPHY, AND FULL WEIGHT-BEARING COMPUTED TOMOGRAPHY

Conventional computed tomography (CT), can provide the surgeon with more information in complex cases, but is not weight bearing. Three-dimensional, weight-bearing cone beam CT, however, does offer three-dimensional imaging while weight bearing, and this is enabling further insight into HV.

For example, traditional radiographic techniques have had problems accurately imaging the sesamoids in HV, for relative displacement and chondral wear. Weight-bearing AP radiographs have been shown to be misrepresentative due to the rotational component to the deformity. Tangential (axial) views overcome this problem; however, to obtain the image, the hallux is placed in a dorsiflexed position (variably between 40° and 75°). It has been shown that the position of the sesamoids varies with the amount of hallux dorsiflexion. Conventional cross-sectional imaging, such as CT and MRI, are not load bearing.[11–13] To overcome these issues, Welck and colleagues[14] investigated the sesamoid position, rotation, and metatarso-sesamoid joint space in a cohort of 43 patients with symptomatic HV compared with a control group of 50 patients using weight-bearing CT scanning (**Figs. 4 and 5**). They found significant differences (*P*<.0001) in sesamoid position, rotation, and metatarso-sesamoid joint space between the 2 groups. In addition, they showed high levels of intra- and interobserver reliability for all measures.

Kim and colleagues[15] also inspected tibial sesamoid position, in relation to first metatarsal pronation in HV patients. They looked at 19 control patients and 138 patients with HV deformities. Using traditional plain radiographs, they found significant differences between the 2 groups in the HVAs and IMAs, as well as significant differences in the first metatarsal pronation angle on semiweight-bearing CT imaging (13.8°, control vs 21.9°, HV). However, there was no correlation between sesamoid apparatus

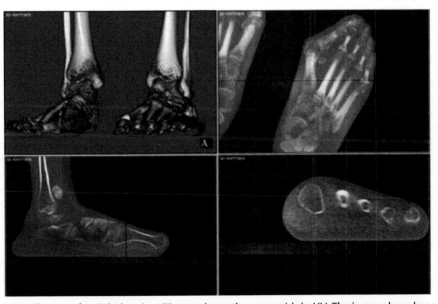

Fig. 4. The use of weight bearing CT to evaluate the sesamoids in HV. The images have been manipulated such that the rotation and position of the metatarsal is standardized and reproducible.

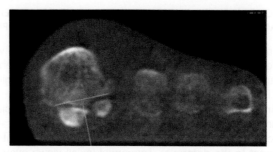

Fig. 5. The measurement of sesamoid position on weight bearing CT. A line was drawn between the lateral edge of the lateral sulcus and the medial edge of the medial sulcus. A perpendicular line was then drawn to the most prominent tip of the crista. The position of the tibial sesamoid relative to this line was noted. (*From* Welck MJ, Singh D, Cullen N, et al. Evaluation of the 1st metatarso-sesamoid joint using standing CT - the Stanmore classification. Foot Ankle Surg 2017;[pii:S1268-7731(17)30059-0]; with permission.)

position and first metatarsal pronation angle, suggesting the latter to be utilized as an independent measurement in HV deformity.

It has also been difficult with traditional radiographic techniques to assess the rotational changes of the metatarsal during weight bearing in HV deformity.[16] These changes are thought to play a crucial role in HV correction.[17] Collan and colleagues[18] investigated, using a portable extremity CT at rest and weight bearing, the rotational position of the first ray, HVA, and IMA in a group of 10 HV patients compared with 5 asymptomatic controls. They found a significant difference ($P<.05$) in the pronation angle of the first proximal phalanx in the HV group compared with the control group ($33° \pm 3°$ vs $4° \pm 4°$ respectively). They also reported significant differences in HVAs and IMAs on weight bearing, but no significant difference of HVAs at rest. There was good correlation between HVAs and IMAs from three-dimensional CT to traditional two-dimensional plain radiographs. The authors highlighted the importance of weight-bearing three-dimensional CT imaging in allowing the surgeon to evaluate fully the deformity in HV prior to corrective surgery.

Kimura and colleagues[19,20] have focused extensively on first ray hypermobility in HV patients using three-dimensional weight-bearing CT. They looked at 10 patients with HV and 10 healthy volunteers. Their results showed, in HV patients compared with controls, significantly greater dorsiflexion at the talonavicular (TN) joint ($P<.05$), significantly greater eversion and abduction at the medial cuneonavicular joint ($P<.05$); significantly greater dorsiflexion, inversion, and adduction at the first tarsometatarsal joint (TMTJ) ($P<.05$); and finally, significantly greater eversion and abduction at the first metatarsophalangeal joint (MTPJ) ($P<.05$, $P<.01$, respectively). Separately they found no correlation between first TMTJ mobility and either the HVA ($P = .78$) or IMA ($P = .11$) in HV patients. Hypermobility of the entire first ray, not only the TMTJ, is an important aspect of HV pathology. Although the magnitude of HV deformity may not correlate with TMTJ mobility, it may be related to other complex joint mobility of the first ray.

Geng and colleagues[21] inspected mobility of the first metatarsal-cuneiform joint in HV and controls during weight bearing using three-dimensional CT. During body weight-bearing conditions, the first metatarsal-cuneiform joint in HV feet dorsiflexed, supinated, and internally rotated to a greater degree than controls. Furthermore, the joint in HV feet widened significantly compared with the controls and tended to translate more in the dorsal-plantar direction.[21] This shows some of the physiologic and pathologic movement at this joint and suggests multidirectional hypermobility at the joint in HV.

MRI

MRI is not routinely performed in the evaluation of HV. However, abnormalities in soft tissue structures such as muscles, tendons, and ligaments contribute to HV deformity progression, as discussed. In this regard, several authors have investigated MRI findings in HV patients. Schweitzer and colleagues[22] recruited 24 patients (11 with HV, 4 with hallux rigidus [HR], and 9 with both HV and HR) who underwent MRI. They observed, in patients with HV, high rates of medial eminence hypertrophy (95%), sesamoid proliferation (90%), sesamoid displacement (83.3%), and the presence of bursa around the first metatarsal head (70%). These findings correlate with those demonstrated on traditional plain radiographs.

Disturbed muscle function and altered tendon positioning are believed to play an important role in HV deformity progression. Eustace and colleagues[23] prospectively studied the MR images of 20 feet with HV and 10 feet without HV to demonstrate tendon shift at the first MTPJ. They reported, in patients with HV compared to those without, the insertion of the abductor hallucis tendon was markedly plantarward; the flexor and extensor hallucis tendons were shifted laterally forming a bowstring, and the sesamoids were laterally rotated within the medial and lateral heads of the flexor hallucis brevis muscle. They found the severity of the tendon shifts to correlate with the HVA and magnitude of clinical deformity. Sanders and colleagues[24] reported on a single case of HV with MRI, which demonstrated lateral displacement of the flexor hallucis longus tendon in relation to the first MTPJ with associated subluxation of the sesamoid bones. The significance of tendons and other soft tissues exerting a deforming force is widely debated with regards to the progression of HV deformity. Indeed, these unfavorable effects may explain the progressive nature of HV and high incidence of postoperative recurrence.

USS

Loss of function of the abductor hallucis muscle is thought to play an important role in the pathomechanics of HV deformity.[25] The abductor hallucis muscle, through isometric contraction, maintains the stability of the first MTPJ and prevents valgus deformity at the MTPJ.[25] With progressive valgus deviation and rotation of the proximal phalanx, the abductor hallucis muscle changes its normal anatomic position, shifting to the plantar aspect of the first metatarsal rather than medial to it, and as such, its function changes from an abductor to a flexor.[25] Stewart and colleagues[26] investigated the characteristics of the abductor hallucis muscle in relation to HV deformity severity using a portable ultrasound system. One hundred two feet with varying severities of HV were categorized into 4 groups according to the Manchester scale[27] (grade 0: no deformity, grade 1: mild deformity, grade 2: moderate deformity, grade 3: severe deformity). Dorso-plantar (DP) thickness, medio-lateral (ML) width, and cross-sectional area (CSA) were measured for each. The authors found significant differences in DP thickness between those with grade 0 (no HV) and grade 2 ($P = .001$) and 3 ($P<.001$), significant difference in ML width between those with grade 0 and grade 2 ($P = .010$), and significant difference in CSA between those with grade 0 and grade 2 ($P<.001$) and grade 3 ($P<.001$). No significant differences were found in any of the muscle characteristics between grades 1, 2, and 3 ($P>.0125$). These findings can be explained by the muscles altered anatomic position in HV feet, resulting in its reduced capacity to function as an abductor. The disuse results in reduced strength and size. As the muscle characteristics do not significantly differ between mild, moderate, and severe HV deformity, it is likely that these changes occur early on in the disease. Preoperative and intraoperative interventions that address abductor hallucis muscle position and function may optimize outcome following HV deformity correction.

INTRAOPERATIVE IMAGING

Another area of development in the imaging of HV is the use of intraoperative fluoroscopy. This is widespread in the field of orthopedic surgery. However, because of radiation legislation and costs, the benefits and risks must be well recognized and documented to justify the use in chosen procedures. Elliot and colleagues[28] investigated whether there is merit in utilizing intraoperative fluoroscopy in HV surgery. They prospectively studied 20 patients undergoing scarf osteotomy HV surgery (28 feet). Intraoperative fluoroscopic images were obtained for all patients with measured parameters to include HVA, IMA, HV interphalangeal (HVIP) angle, and sesamoid position (SES). The images were also analyzed for hardware malposition and complications. The intraoperative imaging findings were correlated with the routine 6-week postoperative weight-bearing plain radiograph findings to determine accuracy and reliability. They found no significant differences in the IMA, HVIP angle, and sesamoid position ($P>.05$) between intraoperative and postoperative images. However, there was a significant increase in the HVA compared with the intraoperative measurements ($4.5°$ to $13.6°$, $P<.001$). This was nevertheless still within normal limits. There were no complications or misplaced hardware revealed by intraoperative imaging, requiring no change to the operative procedure. The authors concluded that intraoperative fluoroscopy is an accurate representation of the 6-week postoperative weight-bearing plain radiographs.

DISCUSSION

Conventional imaging and measurements in HV have problems with reproducibility and accuracy. This is essentially because of the difficulty imaging a multiplanar, three-dimensional deformity, using a two-dimensional imaging modality.

Newer techniques are allowing three-dimensional imaging, while weight bearing, and are starting to add further information on the deformity. For example, more is being learned about the rotational abnormalities and joint instability.

This brings about new challenges and calls for research aiming to work out how best to use these tools, and then validate the techniques for measuring deformity and planning correction. An international research and education initiative named "Weight Bearing CT International Study Group" (ref: https://www.wbctstudygroup.com) was founded in 2016 to tackle these issues.

There is to this date no agreement on the most pertinent way to measure HV deformities in the new, three-dimensional environment. Early research has shown, however, that the technology overcomes the projection and rotation biases related to traditional radiographic setups so that rotation of the foot is more reproducible.[29] Once this is done, the bone axes can be determined using traditional landmarks in the joint, metaphyseal, and diaphyseal regions (**Fig. 6**). Currently, it appears that using the described angles and lengths in a three-dimensional environment requires projections in a two-dimensional plane, thus, reducing the quantity of information, which may miss critical added value rendered available by this technology.[30]

The ability to analyze rotational deformity, such as metatarsal or relative sesamoid rotation in the case of HV, may translate into diagnostic and treatment opportunities.

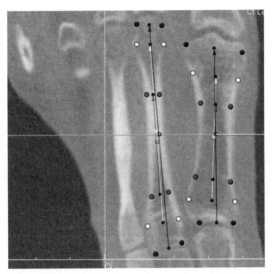

Fig. 6. A demonstration of using the standing CT to measure IMA once foot standardized for rotation. Medial and lateral points of metatarsal at points along the length of the bone (circles).

The question is what to do with this new information or how to relate it to new treatment algorithms.

The answers will come from accumulation and analysis of large quantities of data which require automation and artificial intelligence.

REFERENCES

1. Perera AM, Mason L, Stephens MM. The pathogenesis of HV. J Bone Joint Surg Am 2011;93(17):1650–61.
2. Vanore JV, Christensen JC, Kravitz SR, et al. Diagnosis and treatment of first metatarsophalangeal joint disorders. Section 1: HV. J Foot Ankle Surg 2003;42:112–23.
3. Nix S, Smith M, Vicenzino B. Prevalence of HV in the general population: a systematic review and meta-analysis. J Foot Ankle Res 2010;3:21.
4. Durlacher L. A treatise on corns, bunions and diseases of nails and general management of the feet. London: Simkin, Marshall & Co; 1845.
5. Kilmartin TE, Barrington RL, Wallace WA. Metatarsus primus varus, a statistical study. J Bone Joint Surg Br 1991;73:937–40.
6. Hardy RH, Clapham JCR. Observations on hallux valgus; based on a controlled series. J Bone Joint Surg Br 1951;33-B:376–91.
7. Piggot H. The natural history of HV in adolescence, and early adult life. J Bone Joint Surg 1960;42(4):749–60.
8. Mancuso JE, Abramow SP, Landsman MJ, et al. The zeroplus first metatarsal and its relationship to bunion deformity. J Foot Ankle Surg 2003;42(6):319–26.
9. Coughlin MJ, Saltzman CL, Anderson RB. HV. In: Mann's surgery of the foot and ankle. 9th edition. Philadelphia: Elsevier Saunders; 2014. p. 155–322.
10. Coughlin MJ, Freund E. The reliability of angular measurements in HV deformities. Foot Ankle Int 2001;22:369–79.
11. Kuwano T, Nagamine R, Sakaki K, et al. New radiographic analysis of sesamoid rotation in HV: comparison with conventional evaluation methods. Foot Ankle Int 2002;23:811–7.

12. Smith RW, Reynolds JC, Stewart MJ. HV assessment: report of research committee of American Orthopaedic Foot and Ankle Society. Foot Ankle 1984;5(2): 92–103.

13. Talbot KD, Saltzman CL. Assessing sesamoid subluxation: how good is the AP radiograph? Foot Ankle Int 1998;19(8):547–54.

14. Welck MJ, Singh D, Cullen N, et al. Evaluation of the 1st metatarso-sesamoid joint using standing CT- the Stanmore classification. Foot Ankle Surg 2017 [pii:S1268-7731(17)30059-0].

15. Kim Y, Kim JS, Young KW, et al. A new measure of tibial sesamoid position in HV in relation to the coronal rotation of the first metatarsal in CT scans. Foot Ankle Int 2015;36(8):944–52.

16. Maldin RA. Axial rotation of the first metatarsal as a factor in HV. J Am Podiatry Assoc 1972;62(3):85–93.

17. Scranton PE Jr, Rutkowski R. Anatomic variations in the first ray: part 1. Anatomic aspects related to bunion surgery. Clin Orthop Relat Res 1980;(151):244–55.

18. Collan L, Kankare JA, Mattila K. The biomechanics of the first metatarsal bone in HV: a preliminary study utilizing a weight bearing extremity CT. Foot Ankle Surg 2013;19:155–61.

19. Kimura T, Kubota M, Taguchi T, et al. Evaluation of first-ray mobility in patients with HV using weight-bearing CT and a 3-D analysis system. J Bone Joint Surg Am 2017;99:247–55.

20. Kimura T, Kubota M, Taguchi T, et al. First tarsometatarsal joint mobility in HV: three-dimensional analysis using weight-bearing computed tomography and correlation with degree of deformity. Aofas Annual Meeting, Toronto, June 2016.

21. Geng X, Wang C, Ma X, et al. Mobility of the first metatarsal-cuneiform joint in patients with and without HV: in vivo three-dimensional analysis using computerized tomography scan. J Orthop Surg Res 2015;10:140.

22. Schweitzer ME, Maheshwari S, Shabshin N. HV and hallux rigidus: MRI findings. Clin Imaging 1999;23:397–402.

23. Eustace S, Williamson D, Wilson M, et al. Tendon shift in HV: observations at MR imaging. Skeletal Radiol 1996;25:519–24.

24. Sanders AP, Weijers RE, Snijders CJ, et al. Three-dimensional reconstruction of magnetic resonance images of a displaced flexor hallucis longus tendon in HV. J Am Podiatr Med Assoc 2005;95(4):401–4.

25. Arinci IN, Genc H, Erdem HR, et al. Muscle imbalance in HV: an electromyographic study. Am J Phys Med Rehabil 2003;82(5):345–9.

26. Stewart S, Ellis R, Heath M, et al. Ultrasonic evaluation of the abductor hallucis muscle in HV: a cross-sectional observational study. BMC Musculoskelet Disord 2013;14(45):1–6.

27. Garrow A, Papageorgiou A, Silman A, et al. The grading of HV: the Manchester scale. J Am Podiatr Med Assoc 2001;91:74–8.

28. Elliot RR, Saxby TS, Whitehouse SL. Intraoperative imaging in HV surgery. Foot Ankle Surg 2012;18:19–21.

29. Richter M, Seidl B, Zech S, et al. PedCAT for 3D-imaging in standing position allows for more accurate bone position (angle) measurement than radiographs or CT. Foot Ankle Surg 2014;20(3):201–7.

30. Lintz F, Welck MJ, Bernasconi A, et al. 3D biometrics for hindfoot alignment using weightbearing CT. Foot Ankle Int 2017;38(6):684–9.

Comparison of Three-Dimensional Displacement Among Different Metatarsal Osteotomies

Young Yi, MD[a], Woo-Chun Lee, MD[b],*

KEYWORDS

- Hallux valgus • Three-dimensional displacement • Metatarsal osteotomy

KEY POINTS

- Metatarsal deformity of hallux valgus is a three-dimensional deformity including rotation in coronal plane.
- Theoretically, it is important to understand three-dimensional displacement of the first metatarsal and correct all of the deformities in three dimensions.
- Current methods of metatarsal osteotomy principally try to correct the transverse plane deformity while preserving metatarsal length and avoiding sagittal plane displacement.

INTRODUCTION

Hallux valgus (HV) is a slowly progressing complex three-dimensional biomechanical process. The vertical and horizontal components have been widely explored and are routinely taken into account in the various procedures of surgical correction; the frontal rotation component, in contrast, has been generally overlooked except in a few studies.[1–3] Only pronation of the hallux has been commonly addressed as a common finding in HV. Uniplanar correction on the anteroposterior view of foot would be insufficient, and rotation on frontal plane as well as sagittal alignment should also be well corrected. However, current surgical methods have been developed based on the correction of horizontal plane deformity, which would be inadequate to correct three-dimensional deformity.[4,5] Each metatarsal osteotomy has a different ability to correct the deformity in different planes.

The authors have nothing to disclose.
[a] Department of Orthopedic Surgery, Seoul Paik Hospital Inje University, Joel-Dong 2 Ga 85, Jung-GU, Seoul 100-032, Korea; [b] Seoul Foot and Ankle Center, Dubalo Orthopedic Clinic, Dongjak-Daero 212, Seocho-Gu, Seoul 06554, Korea
* Corresponding author.
E-mail address: leewoochun@gmail.com

THREE-DIMENSIONAL ASSESSMENT OF HALLUX VALGUS DEFORMITY

Weakening of medial soft tissues of the first metatarsophalangeal joint and erosion of the plantar ridge of the metatarsal head between the medial and lateral sesamoids occur early in the progression of HV.

The proximal phalanx drifts into valgus, and the metatarsal head deviates medially as the soft tissues on the medial side become attenuated. Medial deviation of the metatarsal head gives rise to the apparent prominence of the metatarsal head, and a longitudinal groove appears on the medial aspect of the articular cartilage in the metatarsal head.

As the metatarsal head moves medially, the medial sesamoid lies under the eroded metatarsal ridge, so that the lateral sesamoid articulates with the lateral side of the metatarsal head in the first intermetatarsal space.[6,7]

SURGICAL TREATMENT OF HALLUX VALGUS

Surgical options for HV deformity can be classified into metatarsal osteotomy and arthrodesis. Osteotomy may be undertaken proximally or distally. Proximal osteotomies allow a greater correction of the increased intermetatarsal angle than distal osteotomies, which are usually used for mild or moderate deformities. In recent years, diaphyseal osteotomies such as the scarf and Ludloff procedures also have become popular.

On the other hand, the first metatarsophalangeal joint arthrodesis has been used for end-stage osteoarthritis or rheumatoid arthritis patients. The first tarsometatarsal arthrodesis is gaining popularity, because it can correct the intermetatarsal angle or pronation of the first metatarsal bone at its origin. There have been many reports about the outcome of Lapidus surgery. However, controversy over the effective correction of alignment and its maintenance still persists.

Three-Dimensional Consideration for Metatarsal Correction of Hallux Valgus

The procedure should be versatile so that the HVA, the IMA, and the DMAA can be corrected. The procedure should correct the rotation of metatarsal bone in coronal plane, aiming the reduction of the sesamoid bones at the same time. The length of the first metatarsal should be maintained to prevent the development of transfer lesions and metatarsalgia. The dorsiflexion malunion, with the resultant elevation of the metatarsal head, should be avoided. The more complex the shape of the osteotomy line, the stronger fixation stability of 2 fragments. The one with osteotomy taken parallel to the coronal plane has advantages on correction of rotation, but with less fixation stability. The Wider contact area provides the lesser possibility of dorsal malunion.

COMPARISON OF THREE-DIMENSIONAL DISPLACEMENT AMONG DIFFERENT METATARSAL OSTEOTOMIES
Distal Metatarsal Osteotomies

Wilson osteotomy, Mitchell osteotomy, and distal chevron osteotomy are typical distal metatarsal osteotomies (**Fig. 1**). Correction after these 3 osteotomies mainly depends on lateral translation of the distal fragment. These osteotomies allow only minimal rotation.[8,9]

The Wilson procedure

This is an oblique metaphyseal osteotomy from distal medial to proximal lateral, allowing displacement of the metatarsal head laterally and proximally. HV deformity was corrected by lateral translation and angulation of the distal fragment; however,

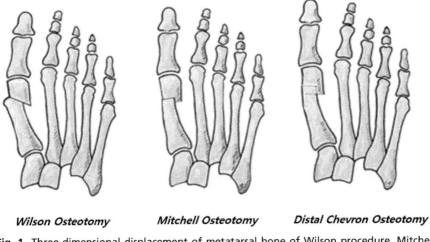

Wilson Osteotomy   Mitchell Osteotomy   Distal Chevron Osteotomy

Fig. 1. Three-dimensional displacement of metatarsal bone of Wilson procedure, Mitchell procedure, and distal chevron osteotomy.

shortening and dorsal translation of the distal fragment occurred as the distal fragment was displaced. Later, Wilson osteotomy was modified as double oblique 45° osteotomy to prevent dorsal displacement of the metatarsal head. Satisfactory results have been described in approximately 90% of patients.[10]

Pouliart, Haentjens, and Opdecam[11] found an average of 8.5 mm shortening of the first metatarsal, and 10 of 32 feet (35%) showed clinically evident shortening of the hallux, which caused extension deformity of the metatarsophalangeal joint. Dorsal angulation was also a common complication that occurred in 7 of 32 feet (26%). Metatarsalgia occurred in 35% of their patients postoperatively and correlated with the amount of shortening. Callosities were present under the second metatarsal head in 78% of their patients. The authors wrote that there were greater amounts of shortening in the presence of metatarsalgia and callosities, but the amount of shortening gives no indication of whether the individual foot will develop metatarsalgia or callosities.[12]

Klosok and colleagues reported mean 10 mm shortening; however, they wrote that the degree of shortening did not correlate with the development of metatarsalgia. Postoperative metatarsalgia was more directly related to insufficient plantar displacement of the first metatarsal head. Double oblique osteotomy helped to maintain plantar displacement to compensate for metatarsal shortening. Despite their modification to make a double oblique osteotomy, elevation of the metatarsal was found radiographically in 20% of their patients.

In summary, Wilson osteotomy achieved correction of hallux valgus deformity by lateral translation and lateral soft tissue relaxation by shortening. The metatarsal head is frequently dorsally translated even with modification as double-oblique osteotomy. Some rotation of the metatarsal head may have been possible as the lateral soft tissue is released; however, there is almost no study about the effect of Wilson osteotomy regarding the rotation in the coronal plane.

The Mitchell osteotomy
This involves a double cut through the first metatarsal neck, leaving a step in the lateral cortex. The capital fragment is displaced laterally and plantarward and held with a suture through drill holes. Good clinical results have been reported with this procedure,

with a 91% rate of patient satisfaction. It is recommended for an IMA up to 15° and HVA up to 35°. Good correction of the deformity has been reported.[13,14]

Nevertheless, shortening of the first metatarsal occurs due to removal of bone to create the step-cut. This, combined with a lack of inherent stability resulting in dorsal malunion, has led to reports of transfer metatarsalgia in between 10% and 30% of patients.[13,15] Loss of correction can also occur. Some authors have reported a decrease in these complications by the use of internal fixation in order to increase stability.[14,16]

In summary, Mitchell osteotomy achieves correction by lateral displacement and shortening of the metatarsal head and shortening of the metatarsal. The metatarsal head is intentionally plantar displaced to compensate for shortening of the metatarsal. Basically, the Mitchell osteotomy is similar to Wilson osteotomy regarding the method of correction of the hallux valgus deformity; however, shortening and dorsal displacement of the metatarsal is less than Wilson osteotomy. Although some rotation may occur during displacement of the metatarsal head, the direction and the degree of rotational correction cannot be consistently and predictably regulated by the operator.

The distal chevron osteotomy

This is a V-shaped osteotomy through the metatarsal neck followed by lateral displacement of the capital fragment. This procedure leads to minimal shortening and is intrinsically stable against dorsiflexion. It is usually indicated for mild-to-moderate deformities.[17]

Excellent clinical results have been reported[12,18] with little or no transfer metatarsalgia when the procedure has been used within limits of correction of the IMA of 4° to 8° and the HVA of 11° to 18°.[12,18] Loss of correction and recurrence can occur from extending the indications to more severe deformities and from loss of position at the osteotomy site. Loss of correction and recurrence can be minimized by cutting technique. The osteotomy with a long dorsal or plantar arm and using internal fixation avoids correction loss.[12,19] However, it can also be employed to correct an increased DMAA by taking a medially based closing wedge to allow medial rotation of the metatarsal head.[12,20] This is termed a biplanar chevron osteotomy. It is treated as a stable osteotomy technique with easy correction, despite showing difficulty of rotation correction on coronal plane.

In summary, chevron osteotomy achieves correction by lateral displacement of the metatarsal head, and addition of medial closing wedge resection is useful for correction of distal metatarsal articular angle. Shortening of the metatarsal and dorsal displacement of the head fragment is less problematic than Mitchell or Wilson osteotomy. Correction in coronal plane cannot be achieved with chevron osteotomy.

Diaphyseal Osteotomies

Ludloff osteotomy and scarf osteotomy are commonly used diaphyseal osteotomies (**Fig. 2**). These osteotomies are done over within the metatarsal shaft and cause anatomic changes in the cortical bone. Therefore, these osteotomies showed high union rate, but they have difficulty in reoperation. Additionally, various three-dimensional changes present around metatarsal bone.[21,22]

The Ludloff osteotomy

This osteotomy consists of a bone cut extending distally and inferiorly from the dorsal cortex, 2 mm distal to the metatarsocuneiform joint, to the plantar cortex.[23] The osteotomy forms an angle of 30° to the long axis of the metatarsal bone. The distal fragment is rotated laterally at the proximal fragment on the coronal plan and stabilized

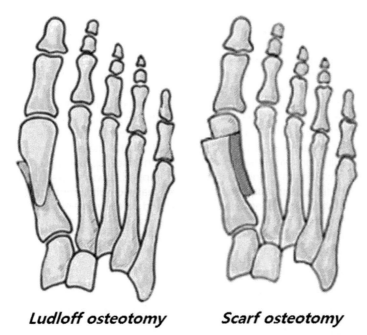

Ludloff osteotomy   **Scarf osteotomy**

Fig. 2. Three-dimensional displacement of metatarsal bone of Ludloff osteotomy and scarf osteotomy.

with 2 screws. It is also possible to displace the metatarsal head plantarwards by the osteotomy technique (oblique osteotomy on the coronal plane). This ensures that elevation of the metatarsal head does not occur and can help relieve pressure on the second metatarsal head. Excellent clinical results have been reported about the Ludloff osteotomy, with good correction of the deformity and without subsequent transfer metatarsalgia.[23,24]

There is minimal shortening of the metatarsal bone, and it is biomechanically more stable than the proximal chevron and proximal crescentic osteotomies.[21,24,25] Variable correction on the transverse plane is not difficult to perform, but trials on metatarsal rotation on coronal plane fall short of expectations.

The scarf osteotomy

This is a Z-shaped step-cut osteotomy named after its woodworking equivalent. A longitudinal cut is made along the length of the diaphysis, sloping plantarward as it passes laterally, allowing plantar displacement and off-loading of the lesser rays. Chevrons are made at each end of the osteotomy to connect it to the dorsal cortex distally and the plantar cortex proximally.

The head and the plantar cortical fragment are then translated laterally, and the osteotomy is stabilized with 2 compression screws. As the technique relies on lateral translation of the metatarsal head rather than angulation on the transverse plane, shortening and increasing in the DMAA is avoided.[21,26]

By altering the geometry of the cuts, it is possible to shorten the metatarsal, or reduce an abnormally elevated DMAA. It can be modified so that an abnormally increased DMAA can be corrected.[27,28] This osteotomy has a high degree of inherent biomechanical stability and is more stable than the basal osteotomies.[29,30]

It is a highly effective and versatile procedure. It has traditionally been recommended for an IMA of up to 18° to 20°[27,31] but by experience can be used for more severe deformities.[26,32,33] The corrective power can be increased by adding a medial closing osteotomy of the proximal phalanx (Akin procedure).

These three-dimensional changes can be determined by the direction of the saw cutting. The obliquity of the bone cutting on the coronal plane of the metatarsal bone affects coronal plane rotation. And the obliquity of bone cutting on the sagittal plane of metatarsal bone affects metatarsal length. A perpendicular osteotomy within the metatarsal bone creates the maximal lateral translation. If the handle of the saw is raised, the first metatarsal head will be depressed, and the metatarsal head will rotate into slight supination, which is desirable. The converse applies with a plane of the osteotomy, in which the handle of the saw is dropped down, whereupon the metatarsal head will tilt up. The result may be a dorsal malunion with pronation of the metatarsal head, associated with an increased likelihood of recurrent HV.[34,35] On the other hand, troughing of the first metatarsal, which occurs as the cortex of the dorsal half of the first metatarsal shaft, collapses and wedges into the softer cancellous bone, leading to pronation and lesser metatarsal overload (**Fig. 3**).[36,37]

Proximal Metatarsal Osteotomies

Proximal wedge osteotomy, crescentric osteotomy, and proximal chevron osteotomy are typical proximal metatarsal osteotomies (**Fig. 4**). Sufficient correction can be obtained and cause a variety of three-dimensional changes, because these osteotomies are located at the proximal metatarsal bone.[21,38]

Proximal wedge osteotomy

An opening wedge osteotomy causes elongation and stretching of the medial soft tissues around osteotomy site and requires a bone graft. It therefore has greater potential for stiffness and nonunion. A closing wedge osteotomy is easier to perform but leads to excessive shortening of the metatarsal.[21,39]

Proximal closed wedge osteotomy has advantage of its concurrent metatarsal valgus angulation and coronal plane metatarsal rotational correction. It is the procedure allowing the most significant angle correction among the metatarsal osteotomies.[21] This osteotomy is inherently unstable, and dorsal malunion occurs in up to 38% of cases, leading to the potential for postoperative transfer lesions.[39] Distraction plates are now available to fix opening wedge osteotomies, and these may improve the results.

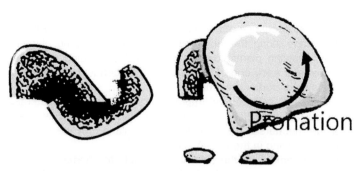

Fig. 3. A diagram illustrates troughing of the first metatarsal, which occurs as the cortex of the dorsal half of the first metatarsal shaft collapses and wedges into the softer cancellous bone, leading to pronation and lesser metatarsal overload.

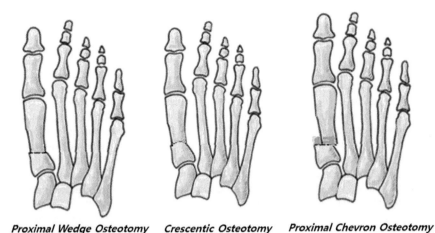

Proximal Wedge Osteotomy   Crescentic Osteotomy   Proximal Chevron Osteotomy

Fig. 4. Three-dimensional displacement of metatarsal bone of proximal wedge osteotomy, crescentric osteotomy, and proximal chevron osteotomy.

The crescentic osteotomy

This osteotomy is widely spread by Mann and Coughlin.[40] It is created 1 cm distal to the metatarsocuneiform joint with a crescentic sawblade and the concavity directed proximally, through a dorsal approach. The metatarsal shaft is rotated laterally, and the osteotomy is held with a lag screw, a Steinmann pin, or multiple Kirschner wires. It leads to minimal shortening of the first metatarsal.

This osteotomy is quite uniplanar procedure on the coronal plane. Therefore, this osteotomy preserves the length of the metatarsal bones. Sagittal correction of the metatarsal bones to the plantar or dorsal side is hard to control, and achieving rotation on the coronal is challenging. However, Lippert and McDermott[38] demonstrated that tilting the saw position obliquely toward the sesamoids results in metatarsal external rotation on the coronal plane in the crescentic osteotomy.

Excellent results have been described, with rates of patient satisfaction of greater than 90% and good correction of the IMA and HVA even in severe cases.[41,42] However, some have found it technically difficult, and its instability has led to dorsal malunion in up to 17% of patients with consequent transfer metatarsalgia.[43,44]

The proximal chevron osteotomy

This is technically easier and intrinsically more stable to dorsiflexion than the crescentic osteotomy. It has been shown to cause less transfer lesions.[44–46] Good results have been described.[3,46]

It involves a medial approach to the metatarsal and creation of a proximally or distally based V-shaped osteotomy. The corrected position is held with a K-wires or a screw.

The proximal chevron osteotomy was a procedure for structural stability. However, as the stable fixation advanced, rather it evolved into a way to try a variety of three-dimensional changes.

A bone graft from the excised medial upper eminence is inserted in the gap for stability, usually after that metatarsal bone placed external rotation on the coronal plane. Conversely, it is possible to technically induce the metatarsal bone internal rotation on the coronal plane.[3,46] The metatarsal bone correction on the sagittal plane affects degrees of elevation of the metatarsal head. There is minimal shortening of the metatarsal bone, and variable correction on the transverse plane and sagittal plane is not difficult to perform surgery.

Arthrodeses

First tarsometatarsal joint arthrodesis (Lapidus)

This is indicated in combination with a distal soft-tissue procedure in the patient with hypermobility of the first tarsometatarsal joint, especially if associated with generalized ligamentous laxity. Mann and Coughlin[40] estimate this to occur in approximately 3% to 5% of patients. Hypermobility can be determined clinically as outlined previously, but it is difficult to estimate accurately and reproducibly.[47] The procedure is also indicated in the presence of degenerative changes on the first or second tarsometatarsal joint and is an option in severe deformity with an IMA of greater than 20°.

The biggest benefit of this procedure is one can perform the correction on the point of the deformity first developed. Furthermore, it is much favorable to correct rotation on the coronal plane, and angular correction to any direction can be performed by osteotomizing on the articular surface together.

It is contraindicated in the adolescent with an open physis at the base of the first metatarsal bone and also in patients with a short first metatarsal bone or degenerative changes in the first metatarsophalangeal joint.

The procedure is technically demanding and associated with a prolonged period of recovery and increased morbidity when compared with metatarsal osteotomies.[47,48]

It also leads to shortening of tarsometatarsal length, and care must be taken to resect as little bone as possible around the tarsometatarsal joint to avoid this drawback. As the varus of the first metatarsal is corrected, the first ray should be plantarflexed slightly to avoid elevation and transfer metatarsalgia. The rate of patient satisfaction varies between 75% and 90%, with fusion rates of approximately 90%.[47–49]

SUMMARY

Profound understanding has to be made upon diverse three-dimensional deformity to make outstanding clinical achievement in HV deformity. If there is a simple varus deformity on metatarsal bone in foot anteroposterior view, simple lateral translation or valgus angulation osteotomy can bring a good result. However, if there exists a malalignment on the sagittal plane or metatarsal rotational deformity on the coronal plane, surgical procedures such as angulation on the transverse and sagittal plane and rotation on coronal plane would be better than a simple lateral translation-valgus angulation osteotomy.

In the authors' experience, careful observation should always be made on sagittal alignment, and choosing the procedure with lower rate of dorsiflexed malunion is also imperative. It is also vital, needless to say, to have thorough knowledge of three-dimensional changes followed by each surgical procedure.

REFERENCES

1. Eustace S, O'Byrne J, Stack J, et al. Radiographic features that enable assessment of first metatarsal rotation: the role of pronation in hallux valgus. Skeletal Radiol 1993;22:153–6.
2. Eustace S, O'byrne J, Beausang O, et al. Hallux valgus, first metatarsal pronation and collapse of the medial longitudinal arch-a radiological correlation. Skeletal Radiol 1994;23:191–4.

3. Borton DC, Stephens MM. Basal metatarsal osteotomy for hallux valgus. J Bone Joint Surg Br 1994;76:204–9.
4. Robinson AHN, Limbers JP. Modern concepts in the treatment of hallux valgus. J Bone Joint Surg Br 2005;87(8):1038–45.
5. Collan L, Kankare JA, Mattila K. The biomechanics of the first metatarsal bone in hallux valgus: a preliminary study utilizing a weight bearing extremity CT. Foot Ankle Surg 2013;19(3):155–61.
6. Mortier JP, Bernard JL, Maestro M. Axial rotation of the first metatarsal head in a normal population and hallux valgus patients. Orthop Traumatol Surg Res 2012; 98(6):677–83.
7. McCarthy AD, Davies MB, Wembridge KR, et al. Three-dimensional analysis of different first metatarsal osteotomies in a hallux valgus model. Foot Ankle Int 2008;29(6):606–12.
8. Robinson AH, Cullen NP, Chhaya NC, et al. Variation of the distal metatarsal articular angle with axial rotation and inclination of the first metatarsal. Foot Ankle Int 2006;27(12):1036–40.
9. Lucijanic I, Bicanic G, Sonicki Z, et al. Treatment of hallux valgus with three-dimensional modification of Mitchell's osteotomy: technique and results. J Am Podiatr Med Assoc 2009;99(2):162–72.
10. Keogh P, Jaishanker JS, O'Connell RJ, et al. The modified Wilson osteotomy for hallux valgus. Clin Orthop 1990;255:263–7.
11. Pouliart N, Haentjens P, Opdecam P. Clinical and radiological evaluation of Wilson osteotomy for hallux valgus. Foot Ankle Int 1996;17:388–94.
12. Nery C, Barroco R, Réssio C. Biplanar chevron osteotomy. Foot Ankle Int 2002;23: 792–8.
13. Kuo CH, Huang PJ, Cheng YM, et al. Modified Mitchell osteotomy for hallux valgus. Foot Ankle Int 1998;19:585–9.
14. Briggs TW, Smith P, McAuliffe TB. Mitchell's osteotomy using internal fixation and early mobilisation. J Bone Joint Surg Br 1992;74-B:137–9.
15. Hawkins FB, Mitchell CL, Hedrick CW. Correction of hallux valgus by metatarsal osteotomy. J Bone Joint Surg Am 1945;27-A:387–94.
16. Blum JL. The modified Mitchell osteotomy-bunionectomy: indications and technical considerations. Foot Ankle Int 1994;15:103–6.
17. Coull R, Stephens MM. Operative decision making in hallux valgus. Curr Orthop 2002;16:180–6.
18. Trnka HJ, Zembsch A, Weisauer H, et al. Modified Austin procedure for correction of hallux valgus. Foot Ankle Int 1997;18:119–27.
19. Donnelly RE, Saltzman CL, Kile TA, et al. Modified chevron osteotomy for hallux valgus. Foot Ankle Int 1994;15:642–5.
20. Schneider W, Knahr K. Keller procedure and chevron osteotomy in hallux valgus: five-year results of different surgical philosophies in comparable collectives. Foot Ankle Int 2002;23:321–9.
21. Nyska M, Trnka HJ, Parks BG, et al. Proximal metatarsal osteotomies: a comparative geometric analysis conducted on sawbone models. Foot Ankle Int 2002; 23(10):938–45.
22. Beischer AD, Ammon P, Corniou A, et al. Three-dimensional computer analysis of the modified Ludloff osteotomy. Foot Ankle Int 2005;26(8):627–32.
23. Chlodo CP, Schon LC, Myerson MS. Clinical results with the Ludloff osteotomy for correction of adult hallux valgus. Foot Ankle Int 2004;25:532–6.
24. Saxena A, McVammon D. The Ludloff osteotomy: a critical analysis. J Foot Ankle Surg 1997;36:100–5.

25. Nyska M, Trnks HJ, Parks BG, et al. The Ludloff metatarsal osteotomy: guidelines for optimal correction based on a geometric analysis conducted on a sawbone model. Foot Ankle Int 2003;24:34–9.

26. Smith AM, Alwan T, Davies MS. Perioperative complications of the Scarf osteotomy. Foot Ankle Int 2003;24:222–7.

27. Kristen KH, Berger C, Steizig S, et al. The SCARF osteotomy for the correction of hallux valgus deformities. Foot Ankle Int 2002;23:221–9.

28. Nyska M. Principles of first metatarsal osteotomies. Foot Ankle Clin 2001;6: 399–408.

29. Popoff I, Negrine JP, Zecovic M, et al. The effect of screw type on the biomechanical properties of SCARF and crescentic osteotomies of the first metatarsal. J Foot Ankle Surg 2003;42:161–4.

30. Newman AS, Negrine JP, Zevovic M, et al. A biomechanical comparison of the Z step-cut and basilar crescentic osteotomies of the first metatarsal. Foot Ankle Int 2000;21:584–7.

31. Crevoisier X, Mouhsine E, Ortolano V, et al. The scarf osteotomy for the treatment of hallux valgus deformity: a review of 84 cases. Foot Ankle Int 2001;22:970–6.

32. Barouk LS. Scarf osteotomy for hallux valgus correction: local anatomy, surgical technique, and combination with other forefoot procedures. Foot Ankle Clin 2000; 5:525–58.

33. Dereymaeker G. Scarf osteotomy for correction of hallux valgus: surgical technique and results as compared to distal chevron osteotomy. Foot Ankle Clin 2000;5:513–24.

34. Larholt J, Kilmartin TE. Rotational scarf and akin osteotomy for correction of hallux valgus associated with metatarsus adductus. Foot Ankle Int 2010;31(3):220–8.

35. Coetzee JC, Rippstein P. Surgical strategies: scarf osteotomy for hallux valgus. Foot Ankle Int 2007;28(4):529–35.

36. Steck JK, Ringstrom JB. Long Z-osteotomy: a review and new modification to correct troughing. J Foot Ankle Surg 2001;40(5):305–10.

37. Murawski CD, Egan CJ, Kennedy JG. A rotational scarf osteotomy decreases troughing when treating hallux valgus. Clin Orthop Relat Res 2011;469(3): 847–53.

38. Lippert FG III, McDermott JE. Crescentic osteotomy for hallux valgus: a biomechanical study of variables affecting the final position of the first metatarsal. Foot Ankle 1991;11:204–7.

39. Zembsch A, Trnka HJ, Ritschl P. Correction of hallux valgus: metatarsal osteotomy versus excision arthroplasty. Clin Orthop 2000;376:183–94.

40. Mann RA, Coughlin MJ. Hallux valgus-etiology, anatomy, treatment and surgical considerations. Clin Orthop Relat Res 1981;157:31–41.

41. Mann RA, Rudicel S, Graves SC. Repair of hallux valgus with a distal soft-tissue procedure and proximal metatarsal osteotomy: a long-term follow-up. J Bone Joint Surg Am 1992;74-A:124–9.

42. Veri JR, Pirani SP, Claridge R. Crescenitic proximal metatarsal osteotomy for moderate to severe hallux valgus: a mean 12.2 year follow-up study. Foot Ankle Int 2001;22:817–22.

43. Brodsky JW, Beischer A, Robinson A, et al. Hallux valgus correction with modified McBride bunionectomy and proximal crescentic osteotomy: clinical, radiological and pedobarographic outcome. Presented at 31st AOFAS Winter Meeting Specialty Day. San Francisco, March 3, 2001.

44. Easley ME, Kiebzak GM, Davis WH, et al. Prospective, randomized comparison of proximal crescentic and proximal chevron osteotomies for correction of hallux valgus deformity. Foot Ankle Int 1996;17:307–16.
45. Acevedo JI, Sammarco VJ, Boucher HR, et al. Mechanical comparison of cyclic loading in five different first metatarsal shaft osteotomies. Foot Ankle Int 2002;23:711–6.
46. Markbreiter LA, Thompson FM. Proximal metatarsal osteotomy in hallux valgus correction: a comparison of crescentic and chevron procedures. Foot Ankle Int 1997;18:71–6.
47. Myerson MD. Metatarsocuneiform arthrodesis for treatment of hallux valgus and metatarsus primus varus. Orthopedics 1990;13:1025–31.
48. Sangeorzan BJ, Hansen ST Jr. Modified lapidus procedure for hallux valgus. Foot Ankle 1989;9:262–6.
49. Coetzee JC, Wickum D. The lapidus procedure: a prospective cohort outcome study. Foot Ankle Int 2004;25:526–31.

Is the Rotational Deformity Important in Our Decision-Making Process for Correction of Hallux Valgus Deformity?

Pablo Wagner, MD[a],*, Emilio Wagner, MD[b],[1]

KEYWORDS

- Hallux valgus • Rotational deformity • proximal metatarsal rotational osteotomy
- Metatarsal pronation • Algorithm • Treatment

KEY POINTS

- Rotational deformity has been very well documented as part of the hallux valgus deformity and as a postoperative recurrence risk factor.
- The rotational correction must be included as part of the hallux valgus treatment algorithm.
- In cases whereby tarsometatarsal instability or osteoarthritis is evident, a Lapidus procedure, correcting the metatarsal pronation, should be the treatment of choice.
- If no fusion is needed, the proximal rotational metatarsal osteotomy is a reliable, stable, and accurate treatment option that combines varus and rotational correction.

INTRODUCTION

Hallux valgus (HV) is a very common deformity affecting a wide age range but mostly middle-aged woman. No literature exists regarding the prevalence of HV deformity, given the evident bias of nonsymptomatic patients who will never visit an orthopedic clinic.

Disclosures Statement: E. Wagner and P. Wagner are paid consultants for Paragon28. R. Melo receives funding for meeting participation from Bioimplantes.
[a] Universidad de los Andes - Hospital Militar de Santiago, Universidad del desarrollo - Clinica Alemana de Santiago, Av. Vitacura 5951, Vitacura, Santiago, Chile; [b] Universidad del desarrollo - Clinica Alemana de Santiago, Av. Vitacura 5951, Vitacura, Santiago, Chile
[1] Present address: Juan de Austria 1521, Las Condes, Santiago 7550502, Chile.
* Corresponding author.
E-mail address: Pwagnerh1@gmail.com

The population that does look for a solution are the ones with pain and some limitations in daily activities given the great toe deformity. These people want a definitive solution for their problem that is, obviously, effective enough so that it will not be a problem anymore. The HV recurrence rate varies between different medium- and long-term studies; but they show a 15% to 20% and even more than a 50% long-term recurrence rate,[1–4] which is unacceptably high. A few recurrence risk factors have been identified, for example, preoperative and postoperative intermetatarsal and HV angle,[5] underpowered technique,[6–9] metatarsus adductus,[10,11] young age,[12] pathologic hyperlaxity, among others. All these factors are well known and should always be a part of the patient-surgeon presurgical discussion. Nevertheless, there is a very important factor that was described more than 20 years ago but is not usually considered: the metatarsal internal malrotation (pronation).

ROTATIONAL DEFORMITY OF THE FIRST METATARSAL

More than a decade ago, Saltzman, Talbot and Walsh[13–17] published a few HV articles describing the metatarsal pronation and sesamoids dislocation, confirming its importance in HV deformity. Ten years ago, Okuda and colleagues[18] published an article in which a round lateral edge of the first metatarsal head (hence, metatarsal pronation) was a recurrence factor for operated HV. The round lateral edge corresponds to the metatarsal condyles that are visible on an anteroposterior (AP) view given the metatarsal internal rotation. Two years later, they published again that sesamoid mal-reduction was a recurrence factor for HV.[19] More studies came in the following years from Japan and South Korea discussing different aspects of this metatarsal pronation and its relationship with the sesamoids mal-reduction. Chen and colleagues[20] showed that postoperative sesamoid malposition had a negative influence on patients' outcomes after HV surgery. Yamaguchi and colleagues[21] showed how the metatarsal pronation could be evaluated analyzing the shape of the lateral edge of the first metatarsal head. Kim and colleagues[22] found that up to 87% of all their HV patients presented with metatarsal internal rotation (lateral round head shape). Finally, the altered distal metatarsal articular angle in an adult HV spontaneously corrects after performing a pure metatarsal rotational correction.[23,24] Therefore, the angled joint surface is only a sign of metatarsal internal rotation and not really a dysplastic sign. Nevertheless, this finding is not valid for juvenile cases, whereby a real head dysplasia exists.

As the reader can interpret, there is a good amount of information that confirms the importance of the rotational deformity in patients with HV; but no significant shift in treatment protocols has been seen in the literature toward correcting the metatarsal internal rotation. The same techniques have been performed for decades by foot and ankle specialists and taught to residents and foot and ankle fellows.

In 2016[25] and 2017,[26] the authors published a surgical technique that corrects metatarsal varus and pronation through an osteotomy. It was called the proximal metatarsal rotational osteotomy. This osteotomy reliably and accurately corrects both deformities (varus and internal rotation); it is performed through a single proximal metatarsal oblique plane osteotomy, achieving any varus correction through rotation. No wedge resection is needed. The only requirement for this osteotomy to work is the coexistence of a metatarsal malrotation (87% of HV cases), given that the coronal deformity can only be corrected through rotation.

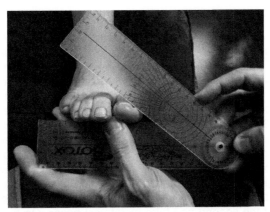

Fig. 1. Nail bed rotation: by using a goniometer, measure the nail rotation in relationship to the foot sole.

Nevertheless, the proximal metatarsal rotational osteotomy has to be carefully planned. The osteotomy obliquity determines the amount of rotation and varus that it will correct; hence, it has to be calculated according to each patient's deformity.

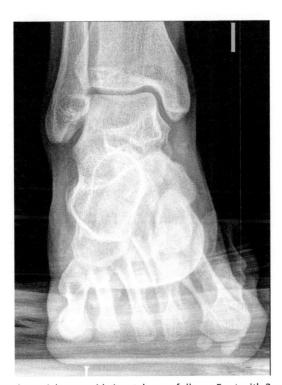

Fig. 2. Weight-bearing axial sesamoid view taken as follows: Foot with 3-cm heel lift, 20° of external rotation, and 20° of toes dorsiflexion. The x-ray cassette is placed behind the heel, parallel to the floor.

PREOPERATIVE WORKUP

Regarding the preoperative analysis for patients with HV, an AP weight-bearing foot radiograph and weight-bearing axial sesamoid views are necessary. The inter-metatarsal angle (IMA) and metatarsal rotation must be measured. The IMA is measured as usual.[26] Metatarsal rotation can be measured in different ways: clinical examination of the great toe/nail bed rotation (using a goniometer, **Fig. 1**), weight-bearing axial sesamoid view (**Fig. 2**), weight-bearing anteroposterior foot radiograph (**Fig. 3**), and weight-bearing computed tomography scan. It is of paramount importance to measure the metatarsal rotation using a weight-bearing image to avoid underestimating the pronation. The way to reliably measure the metatarsal rotation angle in a weight-bearing axial sesamoid view is as follows: measure the angle that results from the intersection of a line that goes between the most medial and lateral ridge of the sesamoid facets and a line drawn on the plantar surface of the second and third metatarsal heads. On the weight-bearing AP foot view, an estimated amount of the metatarsal rotation can be obtained[21] by analyzing the lateral head shape, given that metatarsal head condyles will be more evident with different rotation angles. If an irregular shape on the lateral head can be seen (**Fig. 4**), 10° to 20° of rotation can be safely estimated. If a round lateral head shape can be seen, but a ridge can still be seen on the head, 20° to 30°

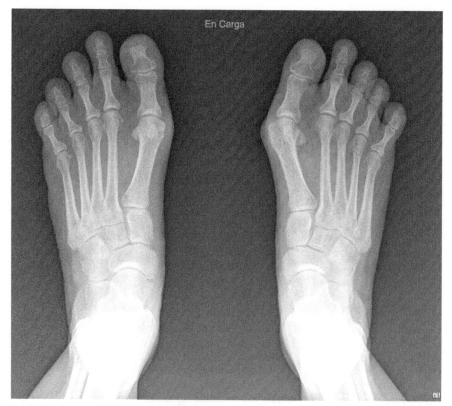

Fig. 3. AP foot weight-bearing radiograph.

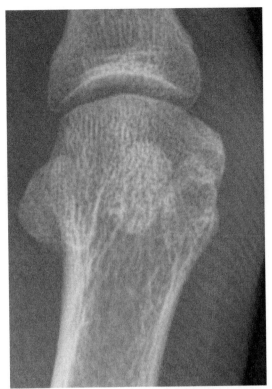

Fig. 4. AP foot weight-bearing radiograph showing a mildly rotated first metatarsal (10°–20°). Lateral head shape (*left side of the image*) is not straight with the metatarsal shaft, showing an abnormal metatarsal rotation. This round edge represents the metatarsal condyles that are visible laterally given the metatarsal pronation.

of rotation can be estimated (**Figs. 5** and **6**). In this case, a perfect circle cannot be drawn around the head that is continuous with the articular surface and lateral head. If a completely round and smooth lateral head shape is evident, with no ridges, 30° or more of rotation is present. In this case, a perfect circle can be drawn following the distal metatarsal articular surface and the lateral head silhouette (**Fig. 7**). Please refer to Yamaguchi and colleagues'[21] study for more details. The sesamoids' position is not a recommended method to measure first ray malrotation.

Another important preoperative aspect to evaluate is the presence of metatarsal instability risk factors and/or radiological signs. The signs are seen on a weight-bearing foot radiograph by looking for a plantar tarsometatarsal joint sag (lateral foot radiograph) or any tarsometatarsal subluxation on the AP view. This finding is not common in the authors' experience in average patients with HV. On the other hand, there are metatarsal instability risk factors, not yet clearly described in the literature, that have been found to be true in the authors' experience. These risk factors comprise young patients (<20 years old) (juvenile HV), hyperlaxity (Beighton score >4), metatarsophalangeal angle greater than 35°, IMA greater than 17°, severe flatfeet, and metatarsal internal rotation greater than 30°.

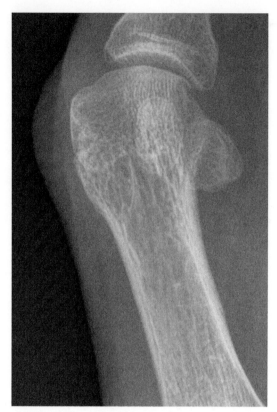

Fig. 5. AP foot weight-bearing radiograph, showing a moderately rotated metatarsal (20°–30°). Lateral head shape (*right side of the image*) is not straight with the metatarsal shaft, showing an abnormal metatarsal rotation. This round edge represents the metatarsal condyles that are visible laterally given the metatarsal pronation.

TREATMENT ALGORITHM INCLUDING ROTATIONAL DEFORMITY

The authors' treatment protocol includes a rotational correction whenever there is a significant (>15°) metatarsal pronation present. Because of the findings already described by Kim and colleagues[22] (dislocated sesamoids in absence of metatarsal rotation), the sesamoids' position should not be a criterion to measure metatarsal rotation. A weight-bearing axial sesamoid view or an AP weight-bearing foot view should be taken to measure the metatarsal rotation. For mild cases with IMA less than 10°, a chevron osteotomy is the procedure of choice regardless of metatarsal rotation. For moderate cases, IMA 11° to 16°, the rotational deformity will define the procedure of choice. If no significant rotation is present, a scarf or proximal oblique sliding closing wedge osteotomy (POSCOW) osteotomy is the authors' recommended surgical technique. If the metatarsal internal rotation is greater than 15°, a proximal metatarsal rotational osteotomy is the authors' preferred technique. For patients with an IMA greater than 17° who are greater than 60 years old, a Lapidus procedure is the recommended procedure. If the IMA is greater than 17°, but patients are less than 60 years old, the proximal metatarsal rotational osteotomy is the authors' recommended procedure. For severe cases (IMA >20°, metatarsophalangeal angle >45°), a Lapidus or a metatarsophalangeal fusion should be

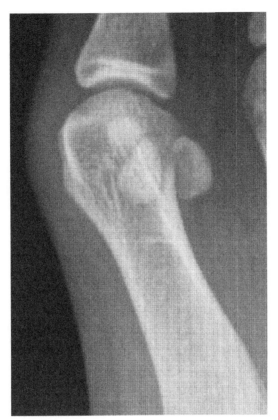

Fig. 6. AP foot weight-bearing radiograph, showing a moderately rotated metatarsal (20°–30°). Lateral head shape (*right side of the image*) is not straight with the metatarsal shaft, showing an abnormal metatarsal rotation. This round edge represents the metatarsal condyles that are visible laterally given the metatarsal pronation.

considered. For all procedures, after the metatarsal correction, an Akin and a bunionectomy are added depending on the cosmetic appearance. A formal lateral release is never performed by the authors' group. Only for severe cases, a lateral transarticular capsular release is performed; but no tenotomies, sesamoidectomies, or ligament elongations are performed.[27] Regarding metatarsosesamoidal osteoarthritis in mild or moderate cases, the authors do not modify their HV algorithm. Symptoms secondary to metatarsosesamoideal osteoarthritis improve after rotational correction, given the redistribution of forces around the joint. For severe osteoarthritic cases, a metatarsophalangeal fusion should be considered.

One of the authors' main concerns is the tarsometatarsal instability. If there are radiological signs of tarsometatarsal instability or arthritis, a Lapidus is the procedure of choice. Before the definitive fixation during the Lapidus procedure, a metatarsal rotational correction should be performed. Sometimes a complete rotational correction is hard to achieve, given the ligamentous constraints, mild arthrosis, capsular adherence, and contractures of a long-standing bunion. The authors do not insist on a complete rotational correction in these cases and are satisfied if 50% or more of the pronation was corrected.

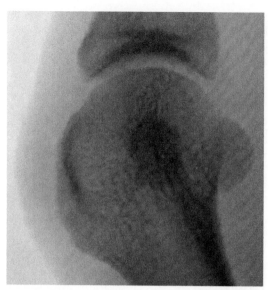

Fig. 7. AP foot weight-bearing radiograph, showing a severely rotated metatarsal (>30°). Lateral head shape (*right side of the image*) is not straight with the metatarsal shaft, showing an abnormal metatarsal rotation. This round edge represents the metatarsal condyles that are visible laterally given the metatarsal pronation. A circle can be easily drawn following the articular surface.

There are cases of metatarsal instability that are discovered (or uncovered) intraoperatively after an osteotomy is performed. The main sign is an HV that recurs intraoperatively after the osteotomy fixation. Bailout options are the following: Convert (if possible) to a Lapidus procedure. Some cases need a fixation to the middle column. Use a screw that extends to the middle cuneiform and/or the second metatarsal base. If the metatarsal osteotomy is already performed, deform the proximal metatarsal segment to its maximum varus deviation. Fix it transiently with a Kirschner wire to the second metatarsal. Then proceed with the osteotomy usual fixation. Perform a definitive fixation of the first metatarsal (proximal to the osteotomy) to the second metatarsal base. This fixation can be performed using a screw or using a suture button fixation (or similar) (**Fig. 8**).

RESULTS

Following the authors' treatment algorithm, they have operated on 25 patients (20 women) with the proximal metatarsal rotational osteotomy technique, with a follow-up of 1 year (9–14 months). The average age was 49 years. They have shown excellent functional results with a lower extremity functional scale score of 58 preoperatively and 73 postoperatively. Postoperative imaging showed a complete rotational metatarsal correction (**Fig. 9**) with an excellent axial alignment. The sesamoids' position changed in all cases from a V or more to a IV or less according to the Hardy and Clapham's[28] classification. No recurrences, complications, or secondary metatarsalgia have occurred in the authors' series. The authors have not observed cases of dorsal malunion or metatarsal shortening.

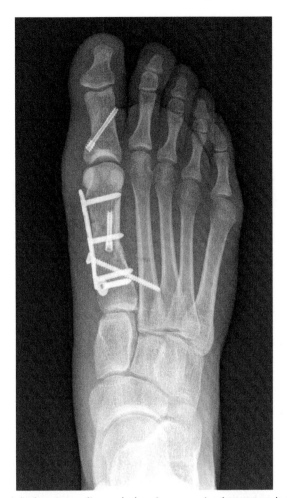

Fig. 8. AP foot weight-bearing radiograph showing a proximal metatarsal rotational osteotomy procedure performed in a patient with unstable HV. A screw was positioned from the first to the second metatarsal base to achieve stability.

SUMMARY

The rotational deformity is a parameter that should be looked for in all HV cases. As already stated, given its importance in functional results[20] and recurrence rate,[18,19] it should be a main part of the surgical treatment.

Correction can be performed through a tarsometatarsal fusion (Lapidus) or through a metatarsal osteotomy. If the former is chosen, classically known as the Lapidus procedure, it can be performed together with rotation of the metatarsal through the joint.[23] This rotation is slightly more difficult to achieve than through an osteotomy, given the ligaments and capsular attachment around the tarsometatarsal joint and given that these patients are older and have an osteoarthritic component to the HV. Lapidus procedures always shorten the metatarsal; hence, metatarsal depression should always be performed to compensate for the shortening and, therefore, try to avoid transfer metatarsalgia. If an osteotomy is chosen, metatarsal supination should be part of the correction capabilities of that technique. To the authors' knowledge, there are

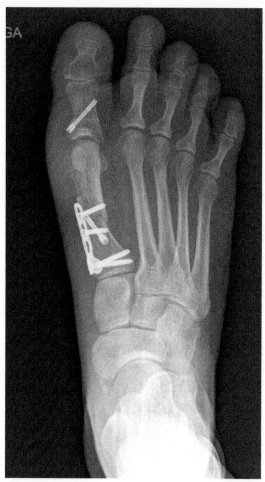

Fig. 9. AP foot weight-bearing radiograph showing a proximal metatarsal rotational osteotomy procedure with a complete rotational and coronal metatarsal correction.

only 3 osteotomies with a supinating ability, the POSCOW,[29] the crescentic osteotomy,[30] and the proximal metatarsal rotational osteotomy.[26] The proximal crescentic is unstable, not frequently used, and has a high rate of dorsiflexion malunion, approximately 20%.[31,32] Metatarsal elevation carries a high risk of HV recurrence and metatarsalgia given the lesser metatarsal heads overload. The proximal metatarsal rotational osteotomy, on the other hand, is an inherently mechanically stable osteotomy because of the proximal-plantar to distal-dorsal bone cut direction (**Fig. 10**). That means that there is a dorsal bone block that prevents the metatarsal from dorsiflexing. In addition, an interfragmentary screw stabilizes the osteotomy together with a medially placed locking plate, which has been proven to be the most stable construct from biomechanical studies.[33,34] The proximal metatarsal rotational osteotomy has another advantage over other proximal osteotomies. It does not resect a wedge of bone to achieve correction. It achieves the deformity correction only through rotation. Therefore, metatarsal shortening is minimal postoperatively, a fact that decreases the risk of metatarsalgia even more. Metatarsal shortening can be accurately performed if

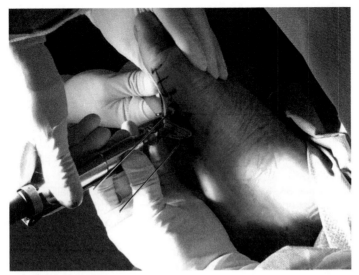

Fig. 10. Intraoperative medial foot view showing the direction of the proximal metatarsal rotational osteotomy, from distal dorsal to plantar proximal.

chosen by the surgeon. Shortening is usually necessary for severe and long-standing HV cases. Usually a 3-mm resection is enough to allow soft tissue relaxation.

Finally, the authors would like to stress the importance that, independent of which technique is chosen, the malrotation is a deformity parameter that must be taken into account if we want to improve our outcomes and decrease the high recurrence rate of our patients with HV. The type of procedure, correction method, and the hardware used are of less importance if the rotation and varus are somehow corrected. It should be taught as a vital part of the HV deformity to new foot and ankle specialists.

REFERENCES

1. Jeuken RM, Schotanus MG, Kort NP, et al. Long-term follow-up of a randomized controlled trial comparing scarf to chevron osteotomy in hallux valgus correction. Foot Ankle Int 2016;37(7):687–95.
2. Bock P, Kluger R, Kristen KH, et al. The scarf osteotomy with minimally invasive lateral release for treatment of hallux valgus deformity: intermediate and long-term results. J Bone Joint Surg Am 2015;97(15):1238–45.
3. Deveci A, Firat A, Yilmaz S, et al. Short-term clinical and radiologic results of the scarf osteotomy: what factors contribute to recurrence? J Foot Ankle Surg 2013; 52(6):771–5.
4. Adam SP, Choung SC, Gu Y, et al. Outcomes after scarf osteotomy for treatment of adult hallux valgus deformity. Clin Orthop Relat Res 2011;469(3):854–9.
5. Okuda R, Kinoshita M, Yasuda T, et al. Hallux valgus angle as a predictor of recurrence following proximal metatarsal osteotomy. J Orthop Sci 2011;16:760–4.
6. Choi GW, Choi WJ, Yoon HS, et al. Additional surgical factors affecting the recurrence of hallux valgus after Ludloff osteotomy. Bone Joint J 2013;95-B(6):803–8.
7. Choi GW, Kim HJ, Kim TS, et al. Comparison of the modified McBride procedure and the distal chevron osteotomy for mild to moderate hallux valgus. J Foot Ankle Surg 2016;55(4):808–11.

8. Crespo Romero E, Peñuela Candel R, Gómez Gómez S, et al. Percutaneous fore-foot surgery for treatment of hallux valgus deformity: an intermediate prospective study. Musculoskelet Surg 2017;101(2):167–72.

9. Fakoor M, Sarafan N, Mohammadhoseini P, et al. Comparison of clinical out-comes of scarf and chevron osteotomies and the McBride procedure in the treat-ment of hallux valgus deformity. Arch Bone Jt Surg 2014;2(1):31–6.

10. Aiyer A, Shub J, Shariff R, et al. Radiographic recurrence of deformity after hallux valgus surgery in patients with metatarsus adductus. Foot Ankle Int 2016;37(2): 165–71.

11. Shibuya N, Jupiter DC, Plemmons BS, et al. Correction of hallux valgus deformity in association with underlying metatarsus adductus deformity. Foot Ankle Spec 2017;10(6):538–42.

12. Agrawal Y, Bajaj SK, Flowers MJ. Scarf-Akin osteotomy for hallux valgus in juve-nile and adolescent patients. J Pediatr Orthop B 2015;24(6):535–40.

13. Saltzman CL, Brandser EA, Anderson CM, et al. Coronal plane rotation of the first metatarsal. Foot Ankle Int 1996;17(3):157–61.

14. Saltzman CL, Aper RL, Brown TD. Anatomic determinants of first metatarsopha-langeal flexion moments in hallux valgus. Clin Orthop Relat Res 1997;339:261–9.

15. Talbot KD, Saltzman CL. Assessing sesamoid subluxation: how good is the AP radiograph? Foot Ankle Int 1998;19(8):547–54.

16. Talbot KD, Saltzman CL. Hallucal rotation: a method of measurement and relation-ship to bunion deformity. Foot Ankle Int 1997;18(9):550–6.

17. Walsh SM, Saltzman CL, Talbot KD, et al. In vivo validation of in vitro testing of hallucal flexor mechanics. Clin Biomech (Bristol, Avon) 1996;11(6):328–32.

18. Okuda R, Kinoshita M, Yasuda T, et al. The shape of the lateral edge of the first metatarsal head as a risk factor for recurrence of hallux valgus. J Bone Joint Surg Am 2007;89:2163–72.

19. Okuda R, Kinoshita M, Yasuda T, et al. Postoperative incomplete reduction of the sesamoids as a risk factor for recurrence of hallux valgus. J Bone Joint Surg Am 2009;91(7):1637–45.

20. Chen JY, Rikhraj K, Gatot C, et al. Tibial sesamoid position influence on functional outcome and satisfaction after hallux valgus surgery. Foot Ankle Int 2016;37(11): 1178–82.

21. Yamaguchi S, Sasho T, Endo J, et al. Shape of the lateral edge of the first meta-tarsal head changes depending on the rotation and inclination of the first meta-tarsal: a study using digitally reconstructed radiographs. J Orthop Sci 2015; 20(5):868–74.

22. Kim Y, Kim JS, Young KW, et al. A new measure of tibial sesamoid position in hallux valgus in relation to the coronal rotation of the first metatarsal in CT scans. Foot Ankle Int 2015;36(8):944–52.

23. Klemola T, Leppilahti J, Kalinainen S, et al. First tarsometatarsal joint derotational arthrodesis. A new operative technique for flexible hallux valgus without touching the first metatarsophalangeal joint. J Foot Ankle Surg 2014;53(1):22–8.

24. Dayton P, Kauwe M, DiDomenico L, et al. Quantitative analysis of the degree of frontal rotation required to anatomically align the first metatarsal phalangeal joint during modified tarsal-metatarsal arthrodesis without capsular balancing. J Foot Ankle Surg 2016;55(2):220–5.

25. Wagner P, Ortiz C, Zanolli D, et al. Hallux valgus treatment. A tridimensional prob-lem. Tobillo y pie 2016;8(2):128–32. Available at: https://www.flamecipp.org/ copia-121-127. Accessed March 2, 2018.

26. Wagner P, Ortiz C, Wagner E. Rotational osteotomy for hallux valgus. A new technique for primary and revision cases. Tech Foot Ankle Surg 2017;16:3–10.
27. Wagner E, Ortiz C, Keller A, et al. Plate position and angular stability: mechanical comparison in sawbone osteotomy models. J Surg Orthop Adv 2013;22(3): 213–8.
28. Hardy RH, Clapham JC. Observations on hallux valgus: based on a controlled series. J Bone Joint Surg Br 1951;33:376–91.
29. Wagner E, Ortiz C, Gould JS, et al. Proximal oblique sliding closing wedge osteotomy for hallux valgus. Foot Ankle Int 2013;34(11):1493–500.
30. Yasuda T, Okuda R, Jotoku T, et al. Proximal supination osteotomy of the first metatarsal for hallux valgus. Foot Ankle Int 2015;36(6):696–704.
31. Schuh R, Willegger M, Holinka J, et al. Angular correction and complications of proximal first metatarsal osteotomies for hallux valgus deformity. Int Orthop 2013;37(9):1771–80.
32. Easley ME, Kiebzak GM, Davis WH, et al. Prospective, randomized comparison of proximal crescentic and proximal chevron osteotomies for correction of hallux valgus deformity. Foot Ankle Int 1996;17:307–16.
33. Wagner E, Ortiz C, Figueroa F, et al. Role of a limited transarticular release in severe hallux valgus correction. Foot Ankle Int 2015;36(11):1322–9.
34. Klos K, Gueorguiev B, Mückley T, et al. Stability of medial locking plate and compression screw versus two crossed screws for Lapidus arthrodesis. Foot Ankle Int 2010;31(2):158–63.

Sesamoid Position in Hallux Valgus in Relation to the Coronal Rotation of the First Metatarsal

Jin Su Kim, MD, PhD[a], Ki Won Young, MD, PhD[b],*

KEYWORDS

- Hallux valgus • Sesamoid position • Metatarsal rotation

KEY POINTS

- Hallux valgus (HV) is not a simple two-dimensional deformity but is instead a three-dimensional deformity that is closely linked to sesamoid position and first metatarsal (MT) pronation.
- HV may or may not be accompanied by sesamoid subluxation and/or first MT head pronation.
- Each of these scenarios should be assessed using weighted computed tomography scan preoperatively, and the necessary corrections should be performed accordingly.

INTRODUCTION

The most important radiologic indices for severity of hallux valgus (HV) deformity are the HV angle (HVA) and the first-second intermetatarsal angle (IMA).[1] HV is classified as mild, moderate, or severe based on the degree of HVA and IMA, and the IMA and HVA are corrected to the normal range after determining the metatarsal (MT) osteotomy site appropriate for each classification.[2] However, these indices are two-dimensional measurements, making them useful for assessment of the correction angle and the degree of HV deformity, but they do not elucidate the actual three-dimensional causes of HV deformity. When treating HV, it is necessary to measure and understand the following three-dimensional deformities to improve the success rate and improve the long-term prognosis. Additionally, one should consider various components or associated disorders of HV in correction of HV.[3]

The first step of deformity correction in the coronal plane is assessment of the degree of sesamoid subluxation and first MT pronation. Previously, sesamoid

Disclosure: The author has nothing to disclose.
[a] Department of Orthopedic, CM General Hospital, 13 Youngdeungpo-ro 36gil, Young-deungpo-gu, Seoul 07301, Korea; [b] Foot & Ankle Clinic, Department of Orthopedic Surgery, Eulji Hospital, 68 Hangeulbiseok-ro, Nowon-gu, Seoul 01830, Korea
* Corresponding author.
E-mail address: youngkw1@hanmail.net

subluxation has been assessed by the position of the sesamoid relative to the first MT shaft on weight-bearing anteroposterior (AP) radiograph, while pronation of the 1st MT was assessed by gross observation of the degree of slanting of the first toenail to the plantar surface.[4] Recently, the three-dimensional sesamoid position has been identified by simple radiographs and computed tomography (CT) scans, and studies have identified the positional relationship between the sesamoid and first MT during walking via weight-bearing CT imaging.

Both sesamoid position and first MT pronation influences the method of HV correction. This article presents a review of the literature addressing the positional relationship of the first MT with the sesamoid, and their clinical significance in relation to three-dimensional deformities of HV.

THREE-DIMENSIONAL DEFORMITY OF THE GREAT TOE IN HALLUX VALGUS

When determining the severity of HV, the IMA is most often used, and most surgeons primarily rely on IMA values for determination of the correction method. However, the IMA measures only a deformity in the transverse plane. Increase of IMA occurs together with axial rotation, or pronation, of the first MT at the TMT (tarsometatarsal) joint.[4-6] The pronation of the first MT causes change in the positions of the abductor hallucis tendon, extensor hallucis longus, and flexor hallucis longus relative to the first metatarsal head. .

With respect to HV deformities, although a larger IMA means a larger DMAA and more severe sesamoid subluxation,[2,7,8] it is necessary to better understand the associations between such deformities.[7] When first MT pronation occurs, the sesamoid appears to be displaced laterally; DMAA is increased, and the lateral side of the first MT head looks round (round-shaped lateral wedge sign) on the foot weight-bearing AP standing radiograph.[9] The stiff intermetatarsal ligament causes pronation of the first metatarsal by holding the lateral sesamoid in its place, as the medialization of the first metatarsal head occurs through the loose medial capsule over the fixed lateral sesamoid.[10] This is referred to as a drive belt sign (**Fig. 1**).[10] Moreover, the morphology of the first MT-cuneiform joint, the degree of hypermobility, the severity of flatfoot deformity, imbalance between the flexor hallucis longus (FHL) and extensor hallucis

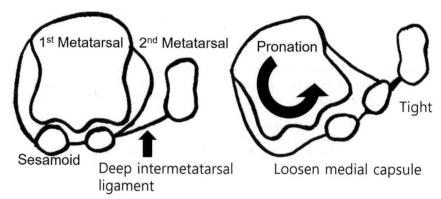

Fig. 1. When hallux valgus occurs, not only does the first metatarsal (MT) move medially on the transverse plane, but rotational deformity in the axial direction occurs as the first MT is pronated. This three-dimensional deformity occurs as the deep intermetatarsal ligament becomes tight, and the medial capsule becomes loose. This is referred to as a drive belt sign.

longus (EHL), weight bearing, and body mass index are also suspected to cause 1st MT pronation deformity.

MEASUREMENT OF SESAMOID SUBLUXATION AND FIRST METATARSAL PRONATION IN HALLUX VALGUS
Measurement of Sesamoid Position from Simple Radiographs

The Hardy and Clapham[11] method of assessing the sesamoid position uses the position of the medial sesamoid on an AP radiograph of the foot. The image was divided into 7 sections relative to the position of the medial sesamoid to the centerline of the first MT, and position 1 of the sesamoid was established as being normal with sesamoid subluxation being graded according to how far medially it was positioned (**Fig. 2**). However, it is difficult to determine the degree of sesamoid subluxation by simple AP weight-bearing radiographs, because this method involves a scale that indirectly expresses the position of the sesamoid and does not show the actual articular surface between the sesamoid and first MT head (**Fig. 3**). A subsequent study found that the distance between the sesamoid and second MT axis remained constant regardless of severity of HV by the first to second intermetatarsal ligament.[12] One should be careful when assessing the degree of sesamoid subluxation on plain radiograph. A tangential sesamoid view that can show the actual articulation of the sesamoid-first MT head was designed, in which radiologic imaging was performed with full dorsiflexion of the great toe (**Fig. 4**). Yildirim and colleagues[13] classified 4 positions of the medial sesamoid relative to the crista (see **Fig. 2**). In grade 0, the medial sesamoid is entirely medial to the intersesamoid ridge; in grade 1, less than a half the width of the medial sesamoid is subluxated laterally. In grade 2, more than half the width of the medial sesamoid is subluxated laterally, and in grade 3, the medial

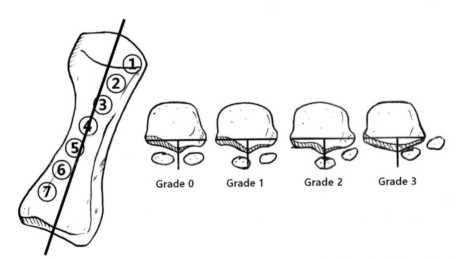

Fig. 2. Method for measuring sesamoid position. (*Left*) Sesamoid subluxation is determined based on the position of the medial sesamoid relative to the centerline of the metatarsophalangeal joint on weight-bearing images. A value of 1 represents a normal position, and 7 represents complete luxation. (*Right*) Sesamoid view image classification. Normal positions are the first MT plantar crista being at the center, medial, and lateral sesamoid positioned in each groove to both sides, and as the first MT is displaced medially, the medial sesamoid does not remain inside the groove and invades the crista. When this becomes severe, luxation can occur.

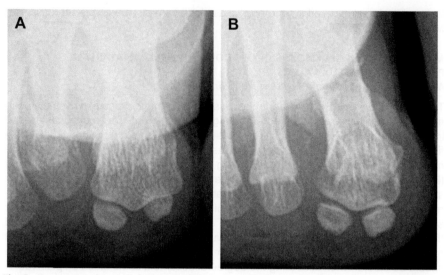

Fig. 3. Tangential views of the sesamoids during weight-bearing (*A*) supination (*B*) prona-tion. The degree of longitudinal rotation of the metatarsal is clearly demonstrated by the position of the sesamoids, which still retain a normal relationship to their facets beneath the metatarsal head.

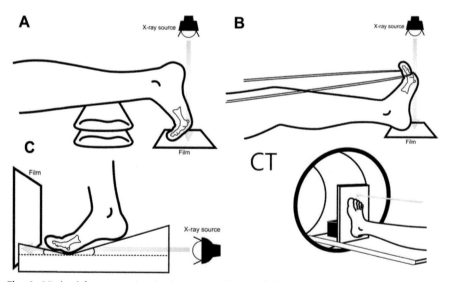

Fig. 4. Method for measuring in the sesamoid view. (*A*) The easiest method of measuring without any tools. The great toe is fully dorsiflexed to check for sesamoid-metatarsal artic-ulation. (*B*) An improved method compared with A, since A may have errors in measuring angles, and the sesamoid view does not have a ground line. This method allows sesamoid luxation and first MT head pronation to be measured relative to the ground with images taken in the same manner each time. (*C*) Acquiring a CT coronal view from a partial weight-bearing CT when a full weight-bearing CT is unavailable. Currently, this is the most accurate method for measuring the characteristics of the first MT.

sesamoid is entirely lateral to the intersesamoid ridge.[13] In this sesamoid view, the articulation of the sesamoid–first MT head, the degree of sesamoid subluxation, and the presence of arthritis all can be assessed directly.

Measurement of Pronation on Simple Radiographs

The method for measuring first MT pronation involves viewing the foot anteriorly during physical examination and measuring the slant of the line drawn vertically from the first toenail.[14] In normal feet with no HV, an average pronation of 7.2° was found, and the first toenail angle increased as IMA increased.[14] This great toe pronation was due to first MT pronation, because when the first MT is pronated, it also causes pronation up to the phalanx connected to the joint capsule. According to a study by Jung,[15] reducing the IMA following proximal chevron metatarsal osteotomy resulted in correction of the interphalangeal angle close to the normal level.

Sesamoid view allows assessment of not only sesamoid subluxation but also axial rotational deformation of the first MT head. However, there may be some inaccuracies in the actual measurements, because there is no reference point. Consequently, some authors have attempted to develop foot plates to allow the sesamoid view to be taken consistently and to insert a metal line in the ground line for accurate measurement of pronation (see **Fig. 4C**).

Scranton and Rutkowski[16] reported that the average first MT pronation in the sesamoid view was 14.5° ± 4° in patients with HV, and they insisted that first MT pronation was originated from rotation of first MT-cuneiform joint.

Simple weight-bearing AP images were used to identify whether first MT pronation was present by checking for rotational deformation of the proximal phalanx and first MT head. The presence of first MT pronation was verified by the round-shaped lateral edge sign reported by Okuda and colleagues,[9] which can be useful in determining the pre- and postoperative correction of pronation (**Fig. 5**). However, Park and Lee[17] reported that round-shaped lateral edge sign is not related to recurrence of HV, and sesamoid position is more effective for prediction of HV recurrence. Measuring the severity of pronation in simple radiographs was difficult, and thus, a preoperative prediction on how much correction was required could not be made.

Importance of Weight-Bearing Computed Tomography

Weight-bearing CT scans are an easier way to measure the rotational status of individual bones, and it may become a valuable research tool in the future.[18] Weight-bearing CT scans provide more information than simple radiographs related to the sesamoid–first MT head complex (see **Fig. 4**; **Fig. 6**).[7,19,20]

Sesamoid view in simple radiographs requires dorsiflexion of the great toe, which generates tension in the flexor hallucis brevis attached to the sesamoid, and, as a result, the dislocated sesamoid is reduced back into its normal position.[13] Consequently, the incidence of sesamoid subluxation may be underestimated. Moreover, an axis is needed for comparison of first MT rotation, but simply bending the toes when acquiring the images makes it difficult to find the changed angle. Moreover, when the patient is walking, the full dorsiflexion used when acquiring sesamoid view images does not occur. Therefore, the clinical significance of the sesamoid subluxation and the first metatarsal pronation on sesamoid view becomes questionable. Recently, full or partial weight-bearing CT scans have been used to check for a sesamoid–first MT complex in weight-bearing status, and the values measured in this manner are used for accurate assessment of first MT rotation and sesamoid subluxation.

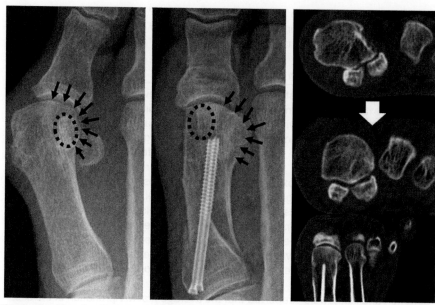

Fig. 5. Checking for the round sign can identify first MT pronation on simple radiographs. When first MT pronation is present (*left*), the medial sesamoid is displaced laterally (*dotted circle*), and the lateral first MT head appears round without forming an angle (*arrows*). However, when the first MT is in its normal position (*middle*), the distal articular margin forms an acute angle and the medial side also forms an angle (*arrows*). Correction for pronation is performed (*right*), and sesamoid subluxation is recovered with the round angle changing to an acute angle.

When the authors have checked the partial weight CT scan, the patient is instructed to gently press the distal resistance board with his or her foot (see **Fig. 4** CT). The coronal axis for assessment of sesamoid subluxation and first MT pronation angle is shown in **Fig. 6**.[7]

Relationship Between Sesamoid and First Metatarsal Pronation on Weight-Bearing Computed Tomography

On weight-bearing CT scans, there are 4 sesamoid positions. Kim and colleagues[7] modified the original tool. On their modified tool, the tibial sesamoid ranged from grade 0 to 3 on the semi-weight-bearing CT axial view (see **Fig. 2**). The first MT pronation angle was evaluated on a semi-weight-bearing coronal CT axial view for the control and study groups.[7]

On axial weight-bearing CT images, the crista area of the MT can be identified by the area with the best view of the sesamoid. Measuring the angle formed by the flat surface (weight-bearing surface) and the line that bisects the dorsal portion of the MT head in the crista area is the most accurate method of measuring pronation in 3 dimensions. This angle is defined as the first MT pronation angle (α-angle, see **Fig. 6**). To obtain the first MT pronation angle, first, an inferior line was drawn between the lateral edge of the lateral sulcus and the medial edge of the medial sulcus. Subsequently, a superior line was drawn between the points of the medial and lateral corners of the first MT head. Second, bisections of the 2 lines were connected to a straight line perpendicular to the horizontal ground axis. Third, the angle was measured between the

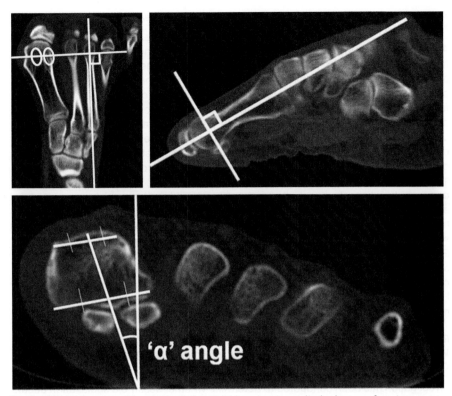

Fig. 6. Weight-bearing CT scan. Partial weight bearing is applied when performing a coronal CT scan in line with the sesamoid axis. For studies of the entire foot, the sesamoid is perpendicular to the third metatarsophalangeal axis, and coronal view images are acquired along that axis and the first MT axis. On the coronal view, the angle formed by the line that connects the crista and the dorsal center of the first MT and the line vertical to the ground line is defined as the first MT pronation angle, which is used to measure 1st MT pronation.

straight line and the vertical line perpendicular to the ground axis that was obtained in the first step (see **Fig. 6**).[7]

In a study by Kim and colleagues[7] that used semi-weight-bearing CT scanning, sesamoid subluxation (more than grade 1 position) was detected in approximately 72% of patients with HV. When comparing simple sesamoid radiographs and CT imaging, a significant correlation was seen in the degree of sesamoid subluxation with a Spearman rho of 0.584, but the measured values differed in approximately 38% of the cases; 25% measured higher, and 13% measured lower. Therefore, caution is required when determining the degree of sesamoid subluxation using the simple sesamoid view. When CT was used to measure the first MT pronation angle, the normal value was 14° on average, whereas the average value for patients with HV was 22°. When the first MT pronation angle was at least 16°, first MT pronation was considered to be more severe than normal, with a 95% confidence interval.[7]

Collan and colleagues[18] used full weight-bearing CT for measurement and reported that the average first MT/ground angle on weight bearing was 18° in healthy people and 21° in those with HV. Future studies are needed to determine whether the first MT pronation angle or the first MT/ground angle would be more clinically helpful.

Sesamoid and Pronation Types Observed Using Weight-Bearing Computed Tomography in Hallux Valgus

According to a study by Kim and colleagues,[7] the tendency for sesamoid subluxation was increased in severe HV cases, while changes in first MT pronation appeared to be independent from the severity of HV. Therefore, when performing correction of HV deformity, first MT pronation must be considered as a separate factor when establishing surgical plans (**Table 1**). If both sesamoid subluxation and first MT pronation are present with HV deformity, plans for correction of each deformity must be established separately. Therefore, the different scenarios were divided into 4 types (**Table 2**). CT 4 positions of at least 1 and less than 1 were defined as S(+) and S(−), respectively, while first MT pronation angles of at least 15.8 °and less than 15.8° were defined as P(+) and P(−), respectively. The most common type was having both pronation and subluxation, which accounted for about 61% of all patients with HV, and patients with more severe HV tended to have both conditions. The next common type was the type with pronation but no sesamoid subluxation, which accounted for 25.9% of cases (**Fig. 7**). Cases with P(+) and S(−) were defined as sesamoid pseudosubluxation, because subluxation seemed to be exist on plain radiograph, but actual sesamoid subluxation did not occur on CT. The incidence of remaining 2 types was small; these were a type of HV without pronation or sesamoid subluxation and another type of HV with sesamoid subluxation but without pronation.

Relationship Between Sesamoid Subluxation or Pronation of the First Metatarsal Versus Amount of Hallux Valgus Angle and Intermetatarsal Angle on Weight-Bearing Computed Tomography Scans

Investigation has been conducted to determine whether sesamoid subluxation occurs more often when HVA and IMA are larger. Sesamoid subluxation becomes more severe as HVA and IMA increase. As the medial sesamoid overlaps the crista, arthritis progresses and arthropathy and joint denudation occur first between the medial sesamoid and crista. In particular, as high-grade HV advances, the grade of arthritis also increases.[20] In the authors' study, a moderate statistical correlation between the CT 4 position and HVA was noted, with a Spearman's rank correlation coefficient rho of 0.477.

The present study investigated whether first MT pronation became more severe as the HVA and IMA increases. In the present study, the first MT pronation angle showed a low correlation coefficient with IMA and HVA, and thus, measurements need to be made separately to determine how the correction should be performed. The fact that HV becomes more severe does not mean first MT pronation also becomes more severe. Therefore, for correction of HV, pronation of the first MT should be

Table 1
Spearman's correlation coefficient between graded measurements

Radiographic Measurements	Spearman's Rank Correlation Coefficient (Rho)
'α' angle vs HVA	0.076
'α' angle vs IMA	0.144
'α' angle vs CT 4 position	0.019
HVA vs CT 4 position	0.477
HVA vs IMA	0.614

Table 2
Determination of surgical plans based on presence of sesamoid luxation and severity of first metatarsal pronation

Type	P(−)	P(+)
S(−)	Transverse osteotomy without lateral release	Supination osteotomy without lateral release
S(+)	Transverse osteotomy with lateral release	Supination osteotomy with lateral release

Abbreviations: P(−), normal first metatarsal pronation angle ('α' angle <16°); P(+), abnormal first metatarsal pronation angle ('α' angle ≥16°); S(−), no tibial sesamoid subluxation (grade 0); S(+), tibial sesamoid subluxation (grade ≥1).

regarded as an independent factor to be corrected. Even a case with a mild HV may have a first MT pronation. Because some authors have claimed that first MT pronation is associated with the severity of HV,[6,21] large-scale follow-up studies on this topic are needed.

However, from a three-dimensional perspective of HV, first MT pronation must be corrected at the same time as IMA and HVA are corrected, and thus, it must be measured individually for each patient. Because a larger first MT pronation angle appears to have a relatively closer relationship with sesamoid subluxation, it can be understood that once first MT pronation occurs, the sesamoid slips and becomes dislocated because of the slope created at first MT head plantar surface in coronal plane (see **Table 1**).

CLINICAL IMPORTANCE
Importance of Understanding the Three-Dimensional Relationship Between Sesamoid and Pronation

When the sesamoid becomes subluxed, the sesamoid-first MT articular contact area becomes smaller, which results in increased pressure and arthritis progression.

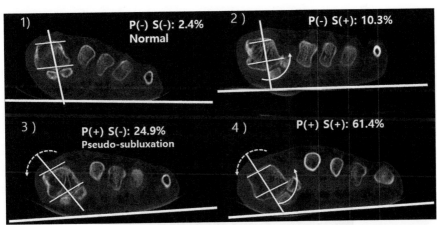

Fig. 7. Four classifications of hallux valgus deformity. (1) P(−)S(−): normal first metatarsal pronation angle (first MT pronation angle<16°) with no tibial sesamoid subluxation (grade 0). (2) P(−)S(+): normal first MT pronation angle (first MT pronation angle<16°) with tibial sesamoid subluxation (grade ≥1). (3) P(+)S(−): abnormal first MT pronation angle (first MT pronation angle ≥16°) with no tibial sesamoid subluxation (grade 0). (4) P(+)S(+): abnormal first MT pronation angle (first MT pronation angle ≥16°) with tibial sesamoid subluxation (grade ≥1).

Moreover, because congruency of the first MTP joint is also lost, arthritis develops in the first MTP joint as well. If the first MT pronation is accompanied with hypermobility, the foot looks like splayed and flat foot. The deformity becomes more severe, and significant arthritic changes can occur on the articular surface between the sesamoid and first MT head.

Clinically, sesamoid reduction and correction of first MT pronation require accurate assessment. Sesamoid subluxation is sometimes not an actual dislocation, and first MT medialization is the primary cause. Therefore, the center of rotation of angulation of the HV should be identified first and the IMA corrected accordingly. If the force holding the adductor tendon is strong, then soft tissue balance should be achieved by lateral soft tissue release and medial capsule plication.[22,23] Moreover, if first MT pronation is present, correction should occur simultaneously. The amount of pronation should be assessed, and supination should be performed during osteotomy for correction to normal position.[7,22,24] Park and Lee[17] reported sesamoid subluxation in immediate postoperative nonweight-bearing foot AP radiograph was 1 risk predictor of HV recurrence during postoperative follow-up. This was also measured from the foot AP radiograph only. Unreduced sesamoid position in AP radiograph should include cases of uncorrected sesamoid subluxation or first MT pronation. Then, one should not decide sesamoid subluxation and first MT pronation by only weight-bearing foot AP radiograph. If you met the sesamoid pseudosubluxation type of HV. Medial capsule plication can be performed by incorrect judgment. It can cause complications because of incongruence of the first MTP Joint (**Fig. 8**).[22]

With HV, it is most common to find cases with both first MT pronation and sesamoid subluxation. However, 12.7% of cases have no pronation, and 28% of cases have no sesamoid subluxation. Therefore, although establishing the correction goals for IMA and HVA may be an important issue for HV correction, attention should also be paid to normalize first MT deformities in the coronal plane. If the sesamoid-MTP joint incongruence or remained first MT pronation angle progress, arthritis and pain may remain when walking after operation.[20,25]

CONCLUSIONS

HV is not a simple two-dimensional deformity but is instead a three-dimensional deformity that is closely linked to sesamoid position and first MT pronation. HV

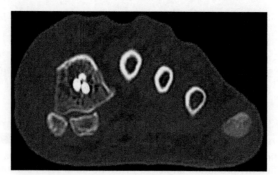

Fig. 8. The severity of first MT pronation and the degree of sesamoid displacement should be accurately assessed prior to surgery to allow alignment to their normal positions during surgery. Excessive soft tissue debridement and suturing after excessive pulling of medial soft tissues results in a poor postoperative prognosis by creating incongruence in the sesamoid-1st MT joint.

may or may not be accompanied by sesamoid subluxation and/or first MT head pronation. Therefore, each of these scenarios should be assessed using weighted CT scan preoperatively, and the necessary corrections should be performed accordingly.

SUMMARY

Weight-bearing CT is an important diagnostic tool to evaluate the three-dimensional relationship between sesamoid and pronation deformity of the HV deformity.

Sesamoid position on simple radiography does not correlate the true subluxation of sesamoid.

Evaluation of the degree of pronation and subluxation of sesamoid is crucial to decide how much to release in lateral structure in addition to the congruity of the first MTP joint.

Surgical attempts to correct pronation should be considered.

REFERENCES

1. Coughlin MJ, Mann RA, Saltzman CL. Surgery of the foot and ankle. 8th edition. Philadelphia: Mosby, Elsevier Inc; 2007.
2. Coughlin MJ, Jones CP. Hallux valgus: demographics, etiology, and radiographic assessment. Foot Ankle Int 2007;28(7):759–77.
3. Dayton P, Feilmeier M, Kauwe M, et al. Relationship of frontal plane rotation of first metatarsal to proximal articular set angle and hallux alignment in patients undergoing tarsometatarsal arthrodesis for hallux abducto valgus: a case series and critical review of the literature. J Foot Ankle Surg 2013;52(3):348–54.
4. Talbot KD, Saltzman CL. Hallucal rotation: a method of measurement and relationship to bunion deformity. Foot Ankle Int 1997;18(9):550–6.
5. Kuwano T, Nagamine R, Sakaki K, et al. New radiographic analysis of sesamoid rotation in hallux valgus: comparison with conventional evaluation methods. Foot Ankle Int 2002;23(9):811–7.
6. Eustace S, O'Byrne J, Stack J, et al. Radiographic features that enable assessment of first metatarsal rotation: the role of pronation in hallux valgus. Skeletal Radiol 1993;22(3):153–6.
7. Kim Y, Kim JS, Young KW, et al. A new measure of tibial sesamoid position in hallux valgus in relation to the coronal rotation of the first metatarsal in CT scans. Foot Ankle Int 2015;36(8):944–52.
8. Dayton P, Feilmeier M, Kauwe M, et al. Observed changes in radiographic measurements of the first ray after frontal and transverse plane rotation of the hallux: does the hallux drive the metatarsal in a bunion deformity? J Foot Ankle Surg 2014;53(5):584–7.
9. Okuda R, Yasuda T, Jotoku T, et al. Supination stress of the great toe for assessing intraoperative correction of hallux valgus. J Orthop Sci 2012;17(2):129–35.
10. Mortier JP, Bernard JL, Maestro M. Axial rotation of the first metatarsal head in a normal population and hallux valgus patients. Orthop Traumatol Surg Res 2012; 98(6):677–83.
11. Hardy RH, Clapham JC. Observations on hallux valgus; based on a controlled series. J Bone Joint Surg Br 1951;33-B(3):376–91.
12. Woo K, Yu IS, Kim JH, et al. Effect of lateral soft tissue release on sesamoid position in hallux valgus surgery. Foot Ankle Int 2015;36(12):1463–8.

13. Yildirim Y, Cabukoglu C, Erol B, et al. Effect of metatarsophalangeal joint position on the reliability of the tangential sesamoid view in determining sesamoid position. Foot Ankle Int 2005;26(3):247–50.

14. Saltzman CL, Brandser EA, Anderson CM, et al. Coronal plane rotation of the first metatarsal. Foot Ankle Int 1996;17(3):157–61.

15. Jung HG, Kim TH, Park JT, et al. Proximal reverse chevron metatarsal osteotomy, lateral soft tissue release, and akin osteotomy through a single medial incision for hallux valgus. Foot Ankle Int 2014;35(4):368–73.

16. Scranton PE Jr, Rutkowski R. Anatomic variations in the first ray: part I. Anatomic aspects related to bunion surgery. Clin Orthop Relat Res 1980;151:244–55.

17. Park CH, Lee WC. Recurrence of hallux valgus can be predicted from immediate postoperative non-weight-bearing radiographs. J Bone Joint Surg Am 2017;99(14):1190–7.

18. Collan L, Kankare JA, Mattila K. The biomechanics of the first metatarsal bone in hallux valgus: a preliminary study utilizing a weight bearing extremity CT. Foot Ankle Surg 2013;19(3):155–61.

19. Lamo-Espinosa JM, Florez B, Villas C, et al. Sesamoid position in healthy volunteers without deformity: a computed tomography study. J Foot Ankle Surg 2016; 55(3):461–4.

20. Katsui R, Samoto N, Taniguchi A, et al. Relationship between displacement and degenerative changes of the sesamoids in hallux valgus. Foot Ankle Int 2016; 37(12):1303–9.

21. Eustace S, Byrne JO, Beausang O, et al. Hallux valgus, first metatarsal pronation and collapse of the medial longitudinal arch–a radiological correlation. Skeletal Radiol 1994;23(3):191–4.

22. Dayton P, Kauwe M, Feilmeier M. Is our current paradigm for evaluation and management of the bunion deformity flawed? A discussion of procedure philosophy relative to anatomy. J Foot Ankle Surg 2015;54(1):102–11.

23. Kim JY, Park JS, Hwang SK, et al. Mobility changes of the first ray after hallux valgus surgery: clinical results after proximal metatarsal chevron osteotomy and distal soft tissue procedure. Foot Ankle Int 2008;29(5):468–72.

24. Dayton P, Kauwe M, DiDomenico L, et al. Quantitative analysis of the degree of frontal rotation required to anatomically align the first metatarsal phalangeal joint during modified tarsal-metatarsal arthrodesis without capsular balancing. J Foot Ankle Surg 2016;55(2):220–5.

25. Suzuki J, Tanaka Y, Takaoka T, et al. Axial radiographic evaluation in hallux valgus: evaluation of the transverse arch in the forefoot. J Orthop Sci 2004; 9(5):446–51.

How I Use a Three-Dimensional Approach to Correct Hallux Valgus with a Distal Metatarsal Osteotomy

Daniel M.G. Winson, MBBS, MRCSEd,
Anthony Perera, MBChB, MRCS, MFSEM, PG Dip (Med Law), FRCS (Orth)*

KEYWORDS

- Metatarsal osteotomy • Minimally invasive technique • Weight-bearing CT

KEY POINTS

- The role of uniplanar osteotomy for the correction of multiplanar deformity in hallux valgus is a developing and promising concept.
- Careful consideration should be given when considering the concept of preexisting pronation of the metatarsal.
- Recent computed tomography studies indicate that there is little or no rotation of the metatarsal itself.
- A multiplanar osteotomy should aim to correct the rotation caused by soft tissue imbalance at the tarsometatarsal and metatarsophalangeal joints rather than in the metatarsal itself.

The concept of metatarsal rotation was established in the 1950s by Hicks.[1] This work was based on the rather rudimentary biomechanical testing available at the time in 5 normal amputated feet. He found that the first ray can move through pronation and supination as it extends and flexes, and abducts and adducts. It is established that this multiplanar movement is present at the tarsometatarsal joints.[2] Although it is likely that other joints also contribute to this overall motion, perhaps to a much greater extent than the first tarsometatarsal joint, with as much as 90% coming through other joints, in particular the navicular cuneiform.[3] However, Hicks' description of total pronation of the first ray of 22° ± 8° was widely accepted.

From this knowledge of the plane of motion of the first ray and the degree of pronation associated with this dorsiflexion and adduction, it naturally led to the assumption

Disclosure Statement: The authors have nothing to disclose.
Trauma and Orthopaedic Department, University Hospital of Wales, Heath Park, Cardiff CF14 4XW, UK
* Corresponding author.
E-mail address: footandanklesurgery@gmail.com

that the first metatarsal head pronates in hallux valgus.[4] Eustace and colleagues[5] investigated this in a number of studies beginning with a cadaveric study in which they found that the plantar tuberosity of the base of the first metatarsal moved laterally (or everted) with closed chain pronation of the foot. Furthermore, they also demonstrated in another clinical study that first ray pronation was intimately associated with medial longitudinal arch height and that it increases with the first ray elevation seen in hallux valgus.[6] This study used weight-bearing radiographs to establish whether the first metatarsal pronates in hallux valgus. By measuring the position of the inferior tuberosity, Eustace and associates were able to show not only that the first metatarsal pronates, but that, as the intermetatarsal angle increases, so does the pronation. They later demonstrated similar findings in MRI investigation of hallux valgus.[7]

More recent studies have also appeared to support these findings. In a study by Mortier and colleagues[8] of weight-bearing radiographs, the mean radiologic pronation was $12.7° \pm 7.7°$ (range, $0°–40°$), although contrary to the findings of Eustace and colleagues there was no correlation M1M2 divergence and pronation. They also found that sesamoid rotation was always found in the presence of pronation, but pronation was not always to be seen with sesamoid rotation, suggesting that sesamoid axial displacement is the root cause of rotational displacement. Mortier and colleagues[8] also performed an anatomic study that showed that very few of the first metatarsals heads were pronated in relation to the base (4 of 20), suggesting that the pronation is at the first tarsometatarsal joint as opposed to metatarsal torsion. However, although this concept has become well-established,[9–17] in Lapidus *The author's bunion*, there was evidence to the contrary.[18] D'Amico and Schuster[19] also showed that the loaded foot did not behave in the manner of the axes reported by Hicks.[1]

The validity of weight-bearing radiographs for measuring rotation had already been called into question by studies using roentgen stereophotogrammetry,[20] and this has been supported with the advent of weight-bearing computed tomography (CT) scans. Collan and colleagues[21] published the findings of the first biomechanical study using weight-bearing CT in hallux valgus. This study compared patients with hallux valgus with a control group in both weight-bearing and non-weight-bearing CT scans. They showed that there was no significant pronation of the first metatarsal but that there was significant pronation of the proximal phalanx ($33° \pm 3°$). Similarly, Geng and colleagues[22] found that most medial cuneiforms pronated more that the first metatarsal and the first tarsometatarsal joint was usually supinated, especially in patients with hallux valgus. Furthermore, Kimura and colleagues[23] demonstrated $4.9° \pm 3.6°$ of supination of the metatarsal relative to the cuneiform at the tarsometatarsal joint and $4.6° \pm 3.4°$ of pronation of the proximal phalanx relative to the metatarsal at the metatarsophalangeal joint. Therefore, the introduction of weight-bearing CT seems to contradict the earlier findings of studies that relied on weight-bearing radiographs in relation to first metatarsal pronation.

The concept that it is the phalanx that pronates is interesting and would correlate with the MRI study conducted by Eustace and colleagues[5] that showed the tendon shift that occurs in hallux valgus. The senior author (AP) described this as subluxation of the hallucal rotator cuff and this results in pronation of the toe.[4] Perhaps this may also result in pronation of the first metatarsal as it slips medially off the sesamoid sling. The rationale for a lateral release is based on reestablishing normal mechanics in this area by releasing the suspensory ligament of the sesamoid and if required the abductor halluces, thus allowing the adductor hallucis to have a stronger effect on the toe (**Fig. 1**A).

The first ray is an inherently unstable array that relies on fine soft tissue balance to maintain its alignment and function fully. The senior author uses a minimally invasive

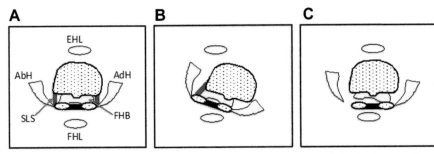

Fig. 1. (*A*) Normal. The hallucal rotator cuff maintains the balance of the fundamentally un-stable axial array of the first ray. (*B*) Hallux valgus before and after surgery. The sesamoid sling subluxes laterally owing to the essential injury to the medial soft tissues. As a conse-quence, the first metatarsal rotates as it slips medially off the pedestal of the sesamoids. The rotation of the tendons changes them into the deforming forces. The SLS is cut and if necessary the lateral head of the FHB and also the AbH. (*C*) This allows the sesamoid sling to come back down under the first metatarsal head. The lateral translation of the metatarsal head along with a derotation allows this to sit back on the sesamoid pedestal and reestab-lish the balance of the tendons. AbH, abductor hallucis; AdH, adductor hallucis; EHL, extensor hallucis longus; FHB, flexor hallucis brevis; FHL, flexor hallucis longus; SLS, suspen-sory ligament of the sesamoid.

approach for hallux valgus that has been previously described.[24] Because this is a closed technique, there can be no reefing of the medial capsule to correct the toe pronation by elevation of the inferior capsule with the attachment of the abductor hal-lucis. Instead, reliance is made on achieving this balance through a combination of soft tissue rebalancing and bony correction in 3 planes to assist achieving and maintaining this rebalancing. We know from the work of Okuda that sesamoid position is very important to the outcomes of the surgery, in reality this is really a surrogate for the position of the hallucal rotator cuff and it is critical that attention is paid to optimizing this.

The first step is a percutaneous lateral release. This technique is performed with a beaver blade passed through the lateral joint from dorsal. The blade is then turned through 90° and brought proximally between the sesamoid and the lateral part of the metatarsal head. This maneuver will release the suspensory ligament of the sesa-moid. The aim is to achieve 10° of passive adduction at the first metatarsophalangeal joint. If this maneuver is not sufficient, then the lateral head of the flexor hallucis brevis tendon attaching to the lateral sesamoid is released by cutting the plantar lateral capsule. If this step is insufficient, then the lateral capsule can be cut, but care must be taken with this cut, because it is a powerful step and can result in overcorrec-tion, particularly in the most severe cases (see **Fig. 1A**).

Next, an osteotomy is performed. The senior author's preference is for a percuta-neous chevron osteotomy performed through a 3-mm incision and using a 2-mm Shannon burr attached to a low-speed, high-torque driver. An extraarticular chevron osteotomy is performed to create a three-dimensional correction.

The use of a uniplanar osteotomy to correct a multiplanar deformity has already been established in both orthopedic surgery such as Blount's correction[25] and more specifically in hallux valgus surgery.[26] Paley[27] tells us that, when rotation and angulation deformities are both present, the axis of rotation and the axis of angulation can be resolved into 1 axis that defines both deformities (**Fig. 2**). In foot and ankle sur-gery, McCarthy and colleagues[26] reported that both Scarf and Stephens basal

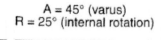

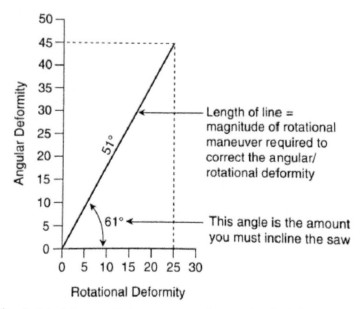

Fig. 2. Calculating multiplanar osteotomies as described by Paley. (*From* Paley D. Radiographic assessment of lower limb deformities. In principles of deformity correction. Springer; Berlin: 2002. pp. 31–60; with permission.)

osteotomies will cause a supination effect and Trnka and colleagues[28] highlight the importance of considering the rotational outcome of a uniplanar osteotomy when performing a Ludloff osteotomy. They demonstrated that a dorsally directed cut will cause pronation, whereas a plantar-directed osteotomy will cause supination.

Of course, these effects are significant for the Scarf and Ludloff osteotomies that include a large degree of rotation. However, the senior author uses these principles to perform a chevron osteotomy with a 2-mm Shannon burr. In the horizontal plane, the burr needs to be angled slightly distally so that it exits 2 mm distal to its entry point to compensate for the width of the bone removal that occurs with a Shannon burr; if lengthening is required the burr is aimed more distally, whereas if shortening is required then the burr is aimed less then 2 mm distally according to the degree required. Similarly in the Coronal plane the burr is aimed at an angle of 10° to 20° relative to the weight-bearing surface of the foot depending on the severity of the deformity to achieve a correction in the coronal and sagittal planes. These 2 planes are linked and it is not possible to correct them independently with this technique.

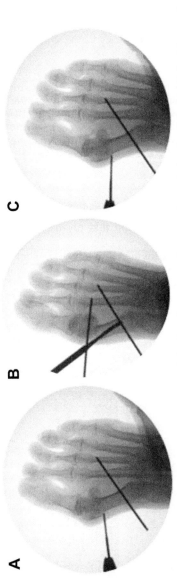

Fig. 3. If the osteotomy is angled at the head/neck junction of the fourth metatarsal a neutral translation is achieved (*A*). In this case, because a Shannon burr has been used for the osteotomy, the osteotomy has to be angled 2 mm further distally to compensate for the bone loss associated with it (*B*). If shortening is desirable, then the osteotomy has to be aimed proximal to the fourth metatarsal head/neck junction (*C*). Lengthening is rarely required and care should be taken with this process, because it can lead to stiffness of the joint.

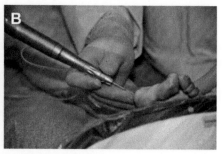

Fig. 4. Axial plane: metatarsal declination and rotation. Because the Shannon burr removes 2 mm of bone, the osteotomy needs to be angled at 10° plantar to the weight-bearing surface of the foot to prevent dorsal translation with lateral translation (*A*). If plantar translation is required, then the burr needs to be angled at more than 10° to the weight-bearing surface, but care must be taken with this maneuver to avoid overplantarization (*B*). Metatarsal head rotation is achieved by the combination of lateral translation and plantar displacement.

Fortunately, there is invariably a need to correct both because the burr also removes 2 mm of bone in the sagittal plane, and first ray elevation is a common finding (**Figs. 3–5**).

The role of uniplanar osteotomy for the correction of multiplanar deformity in hallux valgus is a developing and promising concept. However, careful consideration should be given to the recent literature when considering the concept of preexisting pronation of the metatarsal. These recent CT studies indicate that there is little or no rotation of the metatarsal itself and therefore a multiplanar osteotomy should aim to correct the rotation caused by soft tissue imbalance at the tarsometatarsal and metatarsophalangeal joints rather than in the metatarsal itself.

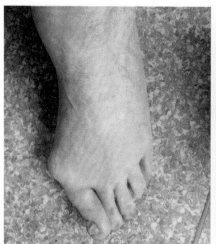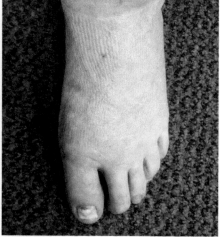

Fig. 5. Preoperative and postoperative photographs of correction of a severe pronation deformity with a minimally invasive percutaneous three-dimensional osteotomy and lateral release resulting in correction of the metatarsal and phalangeal deformity in all 3 planes.

REFERENCES

1. Hicks JH. The mechanics of the foot: I. The joints. J Anat 1953;87(Part 4):345.
2. Winson IG, Lundberg A, Bylund C. Metatarsal motion. Foot 1995;15(2):91–4.
3. Saffo G, Wooster MF, Steven M, et al. First metatarsocuneiform joint arthrodesis: a 5 year retrospective analysis. J Foot Surg 1989;23:191.
4. Perera AM, Mason L, Stephens MM. The pathogenesis of hallux valgus. J Bone Joint Surg Am 2011;793(17):1650–61.
5. Eustace S, O'Byrne J, Stack J, et al. Radiographic features that enable assessment of first metatarsal rotation: the role of pronation in hallux valgus. Skeletal Radiol 1993;22(3):153–6.
6. Eustace S, Byrne JO, Beausang O, et al. Hallux valgus, first metatarsal pronation and collapse of the medial longitudinal arch—a radiological correlation. Skeletal Radiol 1994;23(3):191–4.
7. Eustace S, Williamson D, Wilson M, et al. Tendon shift in hallux valgus: observations at MR imaging. Skeletal Radiol 1996;25(6):519–24.
8. Mortier JP, Bernard JL, Maestro M. Axial rotation of the first metatarsal head in a normal population and hallux valgus patients. Orthop Traumatol Surg Res 2012; 98(6):677–83.
9. Oldenbrook LL, Smith CE. Metatarsal head motion secondary to rearfoot pronation and supination: an anatomical investigation. J Am Podiatry Assoc 1979;69:24.
10. Scranton PE, Rutowski R. Anatomic variation in the first ray: part I anatomic aspects related to bunion surgery. Clin Orthop Relat Res 1988;151:244.
11. Dykyj D. Pathologic anatomy of hallux abductor valgus. In: Clinics in Podiatric Medicine and Surgery. Philadelphia: WB Saunders; 1987. p. 7.
12. Talbot KD, Saltzman CL. Assessing sesamoid subluxation: how good is the AP radiograph? Foot Ankle Int 1998;19:547.
13. McGlamry ED. Hallux sesamoids. J Am Podiatry Assoc 1965;55:693.
14. Olson TR, Seidel MR. The evolution of some clinical disorders of the human foot: a comparative survey of living primates. Foot Ankle 1983;3:326.
15. Grode SE, McCarthy DJ. The anatomical implications of hallux abductor valgus: a cryomicrotomy study 1980. J Am Podiatry Assoc 1980;70:539–51.
16. Roukis TS, Scherer PR, Anderson CF. Position of the first ray and motion of the first metatarsophalangeal joint. J Am Podiatr Med Assoc 1996;86:538–46.
17. Durrant MN, McElroy T, Durrant L. First metatarsophalangeal joint motion in Homo sapiens: theoretical association of two-axis kinematics specific morphometrics. J Am Podiatr Med Assoc 2012;102(5):374–89.
18. Lapidus PW. The author's bunion operation from 1931 to 1959. Clin Orthop 1959; 16:119–35.
19. D'Amico J, Schuster RO. Motion of the first ray: clarification through investigation. J Am Podiatry Assoc 1979;69(1):17–23.
20. Resch S, Ryd L, Stenström A, et al. Measurement of the forefoot with roentgen stereophotogrammetry in hallux valgus surgery. Foot Ankle Int 1995;16(5):271–6.
21. Collan L, Kankare JA, Mattila K. The biomechanics of the first metatarsal bone in hallux valgus: a preliminary study utilizing a weight bearing extremity CT. Foot Ankle Surg 2013;19(3):155–61.
22. Geng X, Wang C, Ma X, et al. Mobility of the first metatarsal-cuneiform joint in patients with and without hallux valgus: in vivo three-dimensional analysis using computerized tomography scan. J Orthop Surg Res 2015;10(1):140.

23. Kimura T, Kubota M, Taguchi T, et al. Evaluation of first-ray mobility in patients with hallux valgus using weight-bearing CT and a 3-D analysis system: a comparison with normal feet. J Bone Joint Surg Am 2017;99(3):247–55.

24. Redfern D, Perera AM. Minimally invasive osteotomies. Foot Ankle Clin 2014; 19(2):181–9.

25. Youngman J, Raptis D, Al-Dadah K, et al. An accurate method of determining a single-plane osteotomy to correct a combined rotational and angular deformity. Strategies Trauma Limb Reconstr 2015;10(1):35–9.

26. McCarthy AD, Davies MB, Wembridge KR, et al. Three-dimensional analysis of different first metatarsal osteotomies in a hallux valgus model. Foot Ankle Int 2008;29(6):606–12.

27. Paley D. Radiographic assessment of lower limb deformities. In: Principles of deformity correction. Berlin: Springer; 2002. p. 31–60.

28. Trnka HJ, Parks BG, Myerson MS. The Ludloff metatarsal osteotomy: guidelines for optimal correction based on a geometric analysis conducted on a sawbone model. Foot Ankle Int 2003;24(1):34–9.

How Do I Use the Scarf Osteotomy to Rotate the Metatarsal and Correct the Deformity in Three Dimensions?

Eric Swanton, MBChB, BA, BHB, FRACS (Orth)[a],
Lyndon Mason, MBChB, MRCS, FRCS Tr&Orth[a,b],
Andy Molloy, MBChB, MRCS, FRCS Tr&Orth[a,b,*]

KEYWORDS

- Hallux valgus • Three-dimensional correction • Rotational osteotomy

KEY POINTS

- The scarf osteotomy has become the workhorse procedure for a large proportion of foot and ankle surgeons, especially in Europe, in the treatment of hallux valgus.
- Such a versatile procedure should not be underestimated, and planning and thought should precede any such procedure.
- The angle of bone cuts and magnitude of translation dictate the final position, and all movement axes should be given equal attention.

INTRODUCTION

The scarf osteotomy is a well-established procedure in the treatment of hallux valgus. A survey of Australian orthopedic surgeons found that greater than 50% would perform a scarf osteotomy for moderate-to-severe hallux valgus (HV) deformities when asked.[1] The earliest mention of a first metatarsal midshaft Z osteotomy in the literature is by Meyer in 1926.[2] This osteotomy was formally given its scarf name by Borrelli and Weil[3] in 1984, who along with Barouk[4] popularized the scarf osteotomy for the treatment of HV. Barouk[5] describes the scarf osteotomy as possessing great versatility, as it can be used to not only provide lateral shift of the first metatarsal, but lower or elevate the metatarsal head, lengthen or shorten the first metatarsal, and even provide axial rotation. The authors use the osteotomy for mild-to-severe HV deformities because of its versatility, from mild to complex cases, and proven results.

[a] Consultant Orthopaedic Surgeon, Aintree University Hospital, Lower Lane, Liverpool L9 7AL, Merseyside, UK; [b] Honorary Clinical Senior Lecturer, Department of Musculoskeletal Biology, University of Liverpool, 6 West Derby Street, Liverpool L7 8TX, UK
* Corresponding author.
E-mail address: andymolloy3@gmail.com

Foot Ankle Clin N Am 23 (2018) 239–246
https://doi.org/10.1016/j.fcl.2018.01.008
1083-7515/18/© 2018 Elsevier Inc. All rights reserved.

Because of the complex three-dimensional osteotomy of the scarf, it is technically challenging with a substantial learning curve. Its versatility, although advantageous, increases the risk of malunion, as axial, sagittal, and coronal plane corrections can be made. The results of scarf osteotomy are generally favorable, characterized by Crevoisier describing an 89% satisfaction rate.[6] However, this positive result does not occur across the board. Coetzee described complications in 47% of cases, with troughing being the major complication (occurring in 35% of cases). Davies and colleagues[7] also found the production of unintentional malunions in a geometric study on scarf osteotomies. A method for reducing this complication was described by Murawski and colleagues.[8] By rotating the scarf, the cortices are no longer purely on cancellous bone as opposed to a traditional scarf. This highlights that when undertaking a scarf osteotomy, planning is paramount. Recognition of the three-dimensional aspects of the osteotomy allows all manner of deformities to be corrected and the potential complications negated.

TRANSLATIONAL CORRECTION AND ITS THREE-DIMENSIONAL EFFECT

A scarf osteotomy reduces the intermetatarsal angle through lateral translation of the metatarsal head. The basic concept to comprehend, however, is that with this translation the movement is in 3 planes, not just one. It is therefore paramount to recognize which bone cuts dictate which plane of movement. This is shown in **Fig. 1** and **Table 1**. This demonstrates that with these cuts, one can achieve from neutral sagittal and coronal displacement to large deformity corrections. Standard practice is to make a Z osteotomy (**Fig. 2**) by producing a longitudinal axial cut starting 5 mm from the dorsal surface of the metatarsal head and moving proximally to the inferior flare of the metatarsal shaft. The author and colleagues have published previously their preferred method of this cut being made with a 10° declination angle to prevent dorsal malunions and subsequent transfer metatarsalgia.[9] The 2 parallel sagittal cuts, 1 distal dorsal the other proximal plantar, are performed as planned on a prior templated radiograph, 90° to the second metatarsal shaft. This ensures length remains

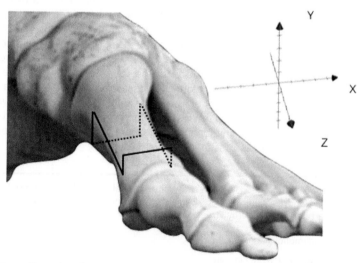

Fig. 1. Three-dimensional representation of a scarf osteotomy illustrating the 3-plane nature of the osteotomy.

Table 1
Bony cuts and the subsequent axis of alteration to which they are attributed

Initial Axis of Movement	Movement	Responsible Bone Cut Angle	Subsequent Axis of Alteration
X	Translation	Horizontal	Y and X
X	Translation	Vertical	Z and X
X	Rotation	Horizontal	Y

Most HV deformities require a translational correction (X axis); however, angulation of the horizontal cut up will result in an elevation of the distal osteotomy limb in the Y axis (ie, elevation of metatarsal head).

unchanged with translation. the authors would therefore consider preoperative templating to be a critical role in the success of this operation.

Using trigonometry, it is possible to predict the 3-plane movement with a translational scarf if one knows the angle of cut (degrees) and magnitude of translation (mm). **Fig. 3** illustrates both the graphs and osteotomy schematic of the expected elevation/lowering/shortening/lengthening of the metatarsal on lateral displacement of the distal limb of the osteotomy. For example, a 6 mm translation of an osteotomized metatarsal with a 30° proximal to distal angulation of both sagittal cuts will result in a 3.5 mm lengthening of the metatarsal. Carr and Boyd proposed 4 mm as an acceptable degree of postoperative shortening,[10] while Schemitsch and Horne[11] concluded that a preoperative relative ratio of the length of the first metatarsal compared with the second of less than 0.825 led to a 50% chance of transfer metatarsalgia in Wilson osteotomies. Karpe reported on the results of shortening scarf osteotomies in severe HV.[12] Although the magnitude of shortening was not reported, it was reported that all patients were satisfied or very satisfied, without any cases of transfer metatarsalgia. The authors standardly template so that there is no change in metatarsal length. However, in the presence of mild arthritis or preoperative

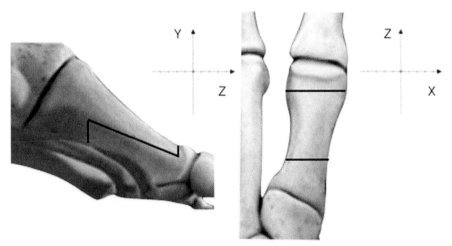

Fig. 2. Example of the typical Z osteotomy performed on the first metatarsal, generally described as a scarf.

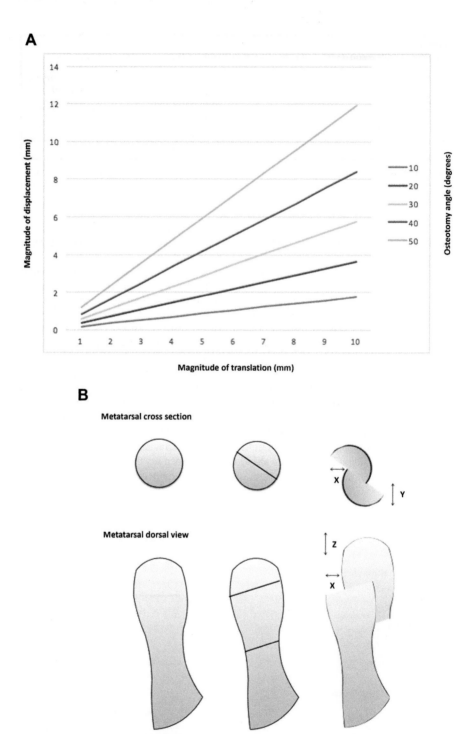

Fig. 3. (A) Graph and (B) schematic illustrating the magnitude of displacement in a particular axis when translated in the juxtaposed axis due to the degree of bony cut. The schematic illustrates the axis.

stiffness, shortening can decompress the first MTPJ and provide a greater arc of movement.

The following section will discuss how each individual plane can be affected with a scarf.

AXIAL ROTATION OF THE METATARSAL HEAD

If an increased distal metatarsal articular angle is to be corrected, a rotational scarf osteotomy in the axial plane is possible where the proximal end of the osteotomy is translated more than distal end. A greater degree of freedom, for an axial plane rotation, is achievable, however, when using a long basal limbed chevron osteotomy.[13] This is because with rotation during a scarf osteotomy, the proximal aspect of the plantar limb can wedge into the dorsal limb, limiting the rotation. In addition, if a significant rotational correction is desired, the proximal end of the plantar limb can abut the second metatarsal, limiting the amount of rotation possible, especially if a particularly long longitudinal osteotomy has been employed. To prevent impaction, a scarf can be modified with a medial wedge of bone excised from the distal dorsal limb, and a small wedge of bone excised from the proximal aspect of the plantar limb. These extra bone cuts result in bone loss, which can inadvertently produce metatarsal shortening. Deenik reported on a randomized control trial comparing scarf and chevron osteotomies for the treatment for HV and found no significant difference in all outcomes. However, they favored the chevron osteotomy, as they considered it to be less technically demanding.[14] The authors concur with this comment when tackling rotational corrections. To help reproducibility, O'Briain and colleagues[15] introduced a formula to control the proximal and distal translations of the osteotomy in a prospective study, improving the distal metatarsal articular angle corrections. An example of use of a scarf osteotomy to correct rotation is illustrated in **Fig. 4**.

ROTATION OF THE METATARSAL HEAD AROUND THE LONGITUDINAL AXIS

The scarf osteotomy was originally designed not to allow metatarsal rotation in the longitudinal axis. However, unintended rotation has been reported as a complication. Davies and colleagues[7] reported a potential risk of producing unintended rotational malunions in all 3 planes. Malunion of the metatarsal in a pronated position has been attributed directly to the effects of troughing in the diaphyseal region of the metatarsal.[16] Two geometric analysis studies have found fewer pronation deformities when comparing scarf osteotomies with other first metatarsal osteotomies. However, these studies were performed in saw bones that would obviously have less susceptibility to trough.[17,18] Murawski recommended some rotation as well as translation of the scarf to prevent troughing, as this gives rise to cortical contact between both limbs of the osteotomy. However, the direction of rotation used in this article would inadvertently increase the distal metatarsal articular angle.[8]

CHANGING LENGTH

Scarf is a wood working technique used in carpentry to increase the length of beams. It is therefore inevitable that its use would be beneficial in lengthening and shortening the first metatarsal. Length can be altered in 2 ways. First, as has already been discussed, the angle of the sagittal cuts relative to the second metatarsal dictates whether the lateral translation will secondarily lengthen or shorten the first metatarsal. Secondly the metatarsal head can be directly translated distally to lengthen or proximally shorten along the longitudinal cut. Defects can be bone-grafted if necessary.

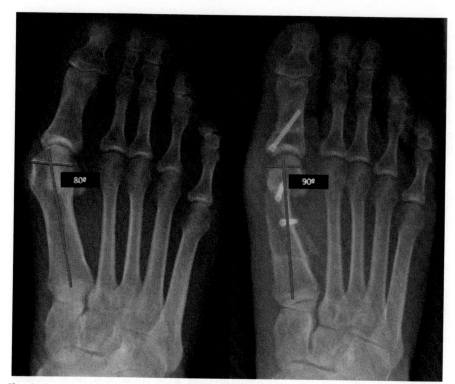

Fig. 4. A preoperative and postoperative anteroposterior radiograph showing the correction of an altered DMAA using a scarf osteotomy.

This method of lengthening was described by Singh and Dudkiewicz for the treatment of iatrogenic first brachymetatarsia.[19] Both lengthening and shortening are easy to plan and control with the scarf osteotomy, as the distraction or shortening by bone cuts can be measured directly due to the gapping between the beams or by the amount of bone removed.

ELEVATION OR LOWERING OF THE METATARSAL HEAD

During a standard scarf, the amount of plantarflexion (lowering) or dorsiflexion (elevation) of the head is controlled by the declination angle of the longitudinal (horizontal) cut. If this is parallel to the floor, then there will be no alteration in metatarsal head height. However, standard practice is to raise one's hand while performing the osteotomy. This causes the metatarsal head to be declined toward the plantar aspect, and therefore, as the osteotomy is translated, the metatarsal head is lowered. The reason for this practice is that HV can defunction the first ray with decreased load being borne by the first metatarsal head. It is therefore apparent that careful planning needs to be undertaken to ensure that the correct degree of lowering of the first metatarsal head is performed.

When using a scarf to lengthen the first metatarsal, Singh and Dudkiewicz modified the direction of the longitudinal cut to be along the axis of the metatarsal. Distal translation here not only achieves an increase in length but also lowers the metatarsal head. If the longitudinal osteotomy is made parallel to the sole of the foot, however, distal translation will not lower or elevate the metatarsal head. These osteotomies can be seen in **Fig. 5**.

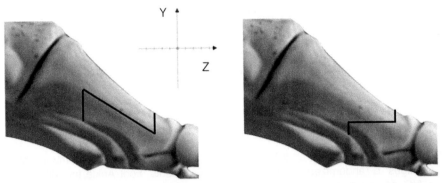

Fig. 5. The initial picture illustrates the scarf osteotomy, which on lengthening would also achieve head declination. If the horizontal aspect of the osteotomy is performed in line with the ground as in the second picture, the metatarsal with lengthen but not decline.

SUMMARY

The scarf osteotomy has become the workhorse procedure for a large proportion of foot and ankle surgeons, especially in Europe, in the treatment of HV. It has predictable results with a meta-analysis of scarf osteotomies for hallux valgus correction finding a mean reduction of 6.21° in the first to second intermetatarsal angle in 300 cases.[20] De Vil[21] reported on the long-term outcomes of scarf osteotomies, with a mean improvement of 1 to 2 IMA of 6° and HVA of 19° being maintained at 8 years. Nevertheless, such a versatile procedure should not be underestimated, and planning and thought should precede any such procedure. The angle of bone cuts and magnitude of translation dictate the final position, and all movement axes should be given equal attention.

REFERENCES

1. Iselin LD, Munt J, Symeonidis PD, et al. Operative management of common forefoot deformities: a representative survey of Australian orthopaedic surgeons. Foot Ankle Spec 2012;5(3):188–94.
2. Meyer M. Eine neue modification der Hallux valgus operation. Zentralbl Chir 1926;53:3265–8.
3. Borrelli AH, Weil LS. Modified scarf bunionectomy: our experience in more than 1000 cases. J Foot Surg 1991;30:609–12.
4. Barouk LS. Scarf osteotomy for hallux valgus correction. Local anatomy, surgical technique, and combination with other forefoot procedures. Foot Ankle Clin 2000; 5(3):525–58.
5. Barouk LS. Forefoot reconstruction. 2nd edition. Paris: Springer-Verlag; 2005.
6. Crevoisier X, Mouhsine E, Ortolano V, et al. The scarf osteotomy for the treatment of hallux valgus deformity: a review of 84 cases. Foot Ankle Int 2001;22(12): 970–6.
7. Davies MB, Blundell CM, Marquis CP, et al. Interpretation of the scarf osteotomy by 10 surgeons. Foot Ankle Surg 2011;17(3):108–12.
8. Murawski CD, Egan CJ, Kennedy JG. A rotational scarf osteotomy decreases troughing when treating hallux valgus. Clin Orthop Relat Res 2011;469(3): 847–53.
9. Molloy A, Widnall J. Scarf osteotomy. Foot Ankle Clin 2014;19(2):165–80.

10. Carr CR, Boyd BM. Correctional osteotomy for metatarsus primus varus and hallux valgus. J Bone Joint Surg Am 1968;50(7):1353–67.
11. Schemitsch E, Horne G. Wilson's osteotomy for the treatment of hallux valgus. Clin Orthop Relat Res 1989;(240):221–5.
12. Karpe P, Killen MC, Pollock RD, et al. Shortening scarf osteotomy for correction of severe hallux valgus. Does shortening affect the outcome? Foot (Edinb) 2016;29:45–9.
13. Favre P, Farine M, Snedeker JG, et al. Biomechanical consequences of first metatarsal osteotomy in treating hallux valgus. Clin Biomech (Bristol, Avon) 2010; 25(7):721–7.
14. Deenik AR, Pilot P, Brandt SE, et al. Scarf versus chevron osteotomy in hallux valgus: a randomized controlled trial in 96 patients. Foot Ankle Int 2007;28(5): 537–41.
15. O'Briain DE, Flavin R, Kearns SR. Use of a geometric formula to improve the radiographic correction achieved by the scarf osteotomy. Foot Ankle Int 2012; 33(8):647–54.
16. Coetzee JC, Rippstein P. Surgical strategies: scarf osteotomy for hallux valgus. Foot Ankle Int 2007;28(4):529–35.
17. McCarthy AD, Davies MB, Wembridge KR, et al. Three-dimensional analysis of different first metatarsal osteotomies in a hallux valgus model. Foot Ankle Int 2008;29(6):606–12.
18. Nyska M, Trnka HJ, Parks BG, et al. Proximal metatarsal osteotomies: a comparative geometric analysis conducted on sawbone models. Foot Ankle Int 2002; 23(10):938–45.
19. Singh D, Dudkiewicz I. Lengthening of the shortened first metatarsal after Wilson's osteotomy for hallux valgus. J Bone Joint Surg Br 2009;91(12):1583–6.
20. Smith SE, Landorf KB, Butterworth PA, et al. Scarf versus chevron osteotomy for the correction of 1-2 intermetatarsal angle in hallux valgus: a systematic review and meta-analysis. J Foot Ankle Surg 2012;51(4):437–44.
21. De Vil JJ, Van Seymortier P, Bongaerts W, et al. Scarf osteotomy for hallux valgus deformity: a prospective study with 8 years of clinical and radiologic follow-up. J Am Podiatr Med Assoc 2010;100(1):35–40.

Using the Center of Rotation of Angulation Concept in Hallux Valgus Correction

Why Do We Choose the Proximal Oblique Sliding Closing Wedge Osteotomy?

Emilio Wagner, MD[a],*, Cristian Ortiz, MD[a], Pablo Wagner, MD[a,b]

KEYWORDS

- CORA • POSCOW • Severe hallux valgus • Proximal osteotomy • Closing wedge

KEY POINTS

- The center of rotation of angulation (CORA) concept relies on determining the apex of the deformity, which allows a complete postoperative realignment.
- Any osteotomy performed outside the apex of the deformity should follow a rule that states that, through displacement and angulation, a realignment will be obtained.
- The proximal oblique sliding closing wedge (POSCOW) osteotomy consists of a proximal closing wedge and chevron osteotomy, combining angulation and translation.
- Future developments in hallux valgus (HV) treatment should center on correcting every plane of the deformity, including coronal and axial components.

INTRODUCTION

Multiple different treatment alternatives exist for HV surgery, and more than 200 different surgeries have been designed. Osteotomies have been recommended for HV surgery for the last 25 years, with good success rates and reliability over time.[1] Generally speaking, distal osteotomies are less powerful and preferred for mild deformities. On the contrary, proximal osteotomies are very powerful to correct large intermetatarsal angles and are the general choice for severe deformities.[2] The recurrence rate of the deformity depends on the preoperative deformity and on the postoperative

Disclosure: The authors have nothing to disclose.
[a] Foot and Ankle Unit, Orthopedic and Traumatology Department, Clinica Alemana - Universidad del Desarrollo, Avda Vitacura 5951, Santiago, Chile; [b] Hospital Militar - Universidad de Los Andes, Avda Alcalde Fernando Castillo Velasco 9100, Santiago, Chile
* Corresponding author.
E-mail address: ewagner@alemana.cl

Foot Ankle Clin N Am 23 (2018) 247–256
https://doi.org/10.1016/j.fcl.2018.01.005
1083-7515/18/© 2018 Elsevier Inc. All rights reserved.

foot.theclinics.com

sesamoid reduction quality, the rate being higher if the HV angle is greater than 37° to 40° and if postoperatively there is an incomplete reduction of the sesamoids.[3–5] Because of these facts, we should obtain, every time, a complete postoperative reduction of the metatarsophalangeal joint and complete correction of the HV deformity. To do this, techniques of variable correcting power are needed.

USING THE CENTER OF ROTATION OF ANGULATION CONCEPT

When planning osteotomies to correct deformities, the principles in deformity correction published some time ago by Paley[6] and Herzenberg prove to be very useful. It is of the utmost importance to be able to determine the center of rotation of angulation (CORA) or apex of the deformity, as it has been named lately in reconstruction literature. In doing so, a proper osteotomy to correct the angulation can be performed.[6] There are 3 general osteotomy rules. Rule number 1 is that the osteotomy that is performed on the apex fully corrects the deformity only through osteotomy angulation. Rule number 2 considers an osteotomy performed away from the apex but achieves complete deformity correction through osteotomy angulation and translation. Rule number 3 consists of an osteotomy performed outside the apex. This osteotomy partially corrects the deformity given that only angulation and no translation is performed through the bone cut.

In HV, if the anatomic axes of the compromised segments are drawn, that is, the proximal phalanx of the hallux, the first metatarsal, and the second metatarsal, it is easy to imagine that there are 2 apices, one distal centered over the metatarsophalangeal joint and one proximal over the naviculocuneiform joint (**Figs. 1** and **2**). No osteotomy can be planned at these sites; therefore, almost every osteotomy will be performed away from the apex of the deformity. Therefore, the osteotomy will follow what is known as the second rule of osteotomies for deformity correction, which states that an osteotomy planned outside the apex of the deformity will correct the alignment but produce a secondary translation. The most commonly performed osteotomy that tries to correct the metatarsophalangeal deformity at the distal apex is the Akin osteotomy. When performing a metatarsal osteotomy that follows the distal apex, unacceptable secondary translation is observed, as exemplified in **Fig. 3**, and a residual deformity due to an increased intermetatarsal angle remains. This incomplete correction explains why most metatarsal osteotomies correct the HV deformity at the proximal apex, and it is the focus of this article.

Distal Metatarsal Osteotomies

Although not perfectly applied, the CORA concept can be exemplified by the commonly used displacement osteotomies, the chevron and scarf osteotomies. These osteotomies correct secondarily the alignment displacing the distal fragment, being limited by the width of the bone. The chevron osteotomy generally achieves 5° of correction, unless displaced more than 40% of the width of the metatarsal head, where contact is significantly compromised, and fixation can only be achieved with Kirschner wires.[7] The scarf osteotomy achieves 5° to 6° of intermetatarsal angle correction,[8] unless modified, increasing the displacement or adding rotation as it has been suggested.[9] Using these modifications, the correcting power of diaphyseal osteotomies can be calculated to be up to 10°, which is not enough to correct severe HV deformities. These data explain why for large intermetatarsal angles, proximal osteotomies are used, achieving large corrections but sacrificing stability, as the fixation of proximal osteotomies is not as reliable as distal osteotomies.

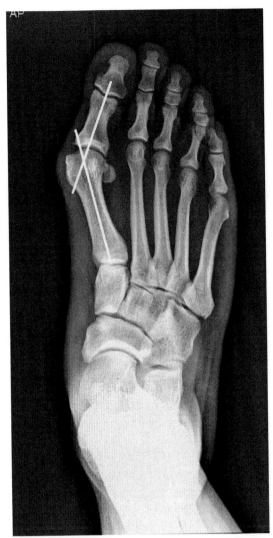

Fig. 1. Radiograph of patient with hallux valgus deformity. Yellow lines represent the proximal phalanx and first metatarsal axes. The intersection of both lines corresponds to the CORA or apex of the metatarsophalangeal deformity.

Proximal Metatarsal Osteotomies

For severe deformities, angular osteotomies have been recommended, as they achieve more correction.[10] Angular osteotomies achieve varus correction in relation to a proximal center of rotation, which immediately confers them an increased correction power in comparison with a distal osteotomy. Nevertheless, by angulating the metatarsal, the distal metatarsal articular angle increases. Some examples of angular osteotomies are the proximal crescentic osteotomy, proximal opening wedge osteotomy, and proximal closing wedge osteotomy. When using displacement osteotomies, like the proximal chevron osteotomy whereby correction is achieved only through lateral displacement, the correction power is limited by the width of the bone, which

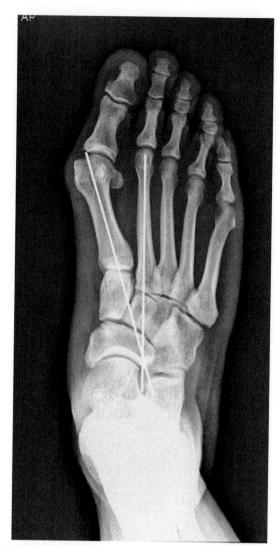

Fig. 2. Radiograph of patient with hallux valgus deformity. Yellow lines represent the first and second metatarsal axes. The intersection of both lines corresponds to the apex of the intermetatarsal deformity.

at the base of the first metatarsal corresponds to approximately 20 mm; therefore, 10 mm of displacement would be considered the maximum translation achievable to keep the bone contact greater than 50%. They correct 1° of intermetatarsal angle per millimeter of lateral translation; hence, they are not very powerful techniques.

In severe deformities, the use of the CORA concept was proposed in 2009 by Mashima and colleagues.[11] In their article, they present their treatment of HV deformity using dome-shaped osteotomies, following more clearly the second rule of osteotomies, which, as stated earlier, achieves correction performing an osteotomy outside the apex of the deformity. The investigators determine 2 different CORAs, one at the metatarsophalangeal joint when analyzing the metatarsophalangeal

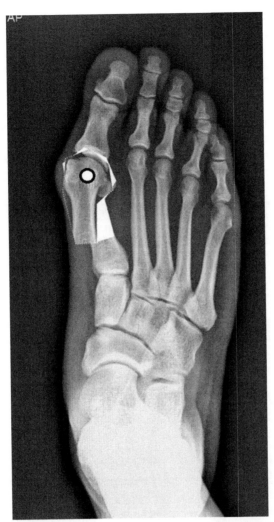

Fig. 3. Preoperative planning of same patient as previous pictures. A simulated proximal os-teotomy is drawn (dotted line), using a distal CORA or apex (black and white circle), achieving correction only through angulation, that is, rule of osteotomy number 3 applies, whereby no translation is performed and a partial correction is obtained.

angulation and a second one on the medial cuneiform when analyzing the intermeta-tarsal deformity. In these cases, the deformity is corrected with a dome-shaped osteotomy on the base of the first metatarsal bone using displacement and angulation, for example, lateral displacement and valgus angulation of the metatarsal bone distal fragment. With this method, complete correction of the deformity in the axial plane is achievable, as the osteotomy can be planned to correct the intermetatarsal angle to 0° if preferred. The final correction and adjustment is done in the operating room using fluoroscopy.

In order to improve the technique, to allow precise preoperative planning, and to make it a more reliable surgical procedure, the idea of the proximal oblique sliding closing wedge (POSCOW) osteotomy was developed.

Proximal Oblique Sliding Closing Wedge Osteotomy

In the authors' opinion, the most important apex in HV cases is the intersection of the intermetatarsal angle. This apex is usually located proximal to the metatarsals, at the level of the navicular and middle cuneiform approximately (see **Fig. 2**). Given that the surgical procedure will be performed on the metatarsal, that is, away from the deformity apex, certain rules have to be followed when developing the POSCOW technique. The POSCOW osteotomy was developed to correct the intermetatarsal angle following the osteotomy rule number 2 and avoiding rule number 3. This idea means that angulation and translation must be combined, given that the procedure is performed away from the apex (**Fig. 4**).

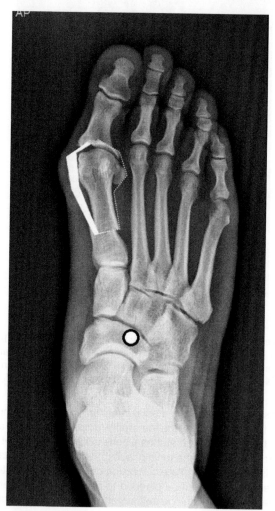

Fig. 4. Preoperative planning of same patient as previous pictures. A simulated proximal osteotomy is drawn (dotted line), using a proximal CORA or apex (black and white circle), achieving correction through angulation and translation, that is, rule of osteotomy number 2 applies, achieving complete correction.

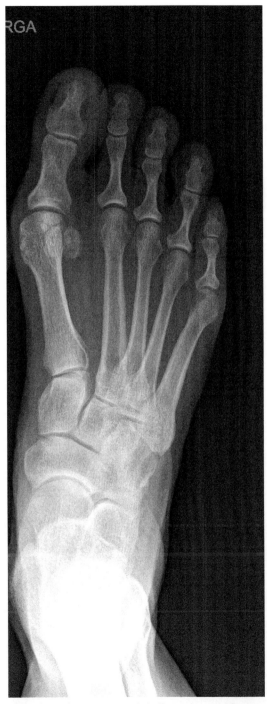

Fig. 5. Preoperative example of a patient with hallux valgus, with a severe deformity.

The POSCOW is defined as a proximal metatarsal osteotomy perpendicular to the long axis of the bone in all planes. A laterally based bone wedge is then removed from the distal fragment, leaving the distal metatarsal segment parallel to the second metatarsal, partially correcting the intermetatarsal angle. Finally, to achieve a complete correction and following the osteotomy rule number 2, a distal fragment lateral displacement is added, achieving a complete correction of the intermetatarsal angle without further increasing the distal metatarsal articular angle (**Figs. 5** and **6**).[12] Performing rotation and displacement achieves a complete deformity correction because it provides a proximal center of rotation, follows rule number 2, and is the key for success in proximal or diaphyseal osteotomies. The POSCOW technique can be

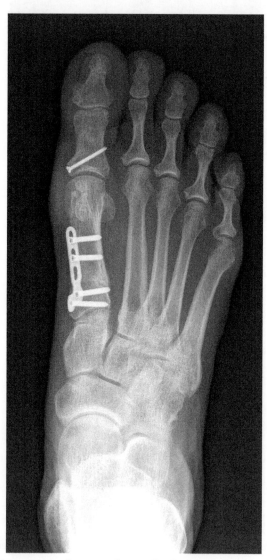

Fig. 6. Postoperative example of same patient as **Fig. 5**, after performing a POSCOW osteotomy, achieving correction through translation and angulation.

understood as a modification of a lateral closing wedge osteotomy with added lateral displacement of the distal segment (ie, proximal chevron effect) along the inclined plane of the initial osteotomy. Based on the mathematical model that was developed,[12] the amount of closing wedge to be resected can be calculated. Noting that a 0.4-mm closing wedge corrects 1° of intermetatarsal angulation (4 mm corrects 10°) and that a 5-mm slide on a 30° inclined plane corrects 4°, we can determine the exact wedge needed to correct the deformity (see **Fig. 4**). The authors published their results on 144 patients (187 feet) who had undergone an operation between May 2005 and June 2010; the median age was 60 years (range, 14–81 years), and the median follow-up was 35 months (range, 12–73). The patient satisfaction rate was 87%. The mean postoperative HV angle was 12.3°, with 24.0° of improvement (range 0–46) ($P<.05$). The mean postoperative IMTT angle was 4.8°, with 10.5° of improvement (range 0–23) ($P<.05$). The mean decrease in the first metatarsal length was 2.2 mm (range 0–8). The mean postoperative American Orthopedic Foot and Ankle Society score was 86 points (range, 25–100) ($P<.05$). Fifteen feet (8%) developed a mild recurrence of HV deformity requiring no treatment, and 12 feet (6.4%) with recurrence of the deformity required revision surgeries.

SUMMARY

Using the CORA concept for any deformity ensures a complete deformity correction. A usual mistake is to forget about rule number 2 whereby a combination of angulation and translation has to be performed on an osteotomy outside the deformity apex in order to achieve full angular correction. This correction is successfully achieved with the POSCOW technique, being able to obtain a complete intermetatarsal angle correction, with no increase in the distal metatarsal articular angle.

In the last few years, the idea of analyzing HV deformity as a multi-planar deformity has been emphasized, adding to the common analysis of varus angulation of the first metatarsal the concept of coronal malalignment, that is, the pronation deformity of the hallux. In 2015, Kim and colleagues[13] described that up to 87% of HV cases had a pronated first metatarsal bone, and 25% of the cases showed an abnormal metatarsal pronation without any sesamoid deviation from its facet. The shape of the lateral edge of the first metatarsal has been found to change depending on the rotation and inclination of the first metatarsal, thereby constituting a good radiological sign of metatarsal pronation.[14] Until recently, the only two techniques that could provide a reliable correction of the pronation of the first metatarsal were a tarsometatarsal arthrodesis, whereby after preparing the joint any desired rotation can be achieved, and any proximal osteotomy whereby a transverse cut was made. When performing a tarsometatarsal arthrodesis, the supination performed on the metatarsal averages 22° as reported by Dayton and colleagues.[15] The POSCOW osteotomy allows varus, translation, and pronation deformity correction through the osteotomy, thanks to its transverse orientation. Nevertheless, no precise measure of the rotation needed is available, and the correction is performed freehand using fluoroscopy to control it. The only available technique that considers the rotation deformity of the first metatarsal and the varus angulation at the same time, precisely correcting the multi-planar deformity, is the PROMO technique.[16]

In summary, using the CORA concept in correcting HV deformity allows the surgeon to accurately measure the deformity and perform more precise osteotomies, which will produce angulation and displacement, allowing a complete realignment of the bone axes. The authors think that the future direction of HV correction relies on considering the deformity as a multi-planar one, adding to the armamentarium techniques that can also correct the coronal deformity, a component that has been overlooked for decades and has only recently gained attention from the orthopedic community.

REFERENCES

1. Trnka H-J. Osteotomies for hallux valgus correction. Foot Ankle Clin N Am 2005; 10:15–33.
2. Easley ME, Trnka HJ. Current concepts review: hallux valgus part II: operative treatment. Foot Ankle Int 2007;28(6):748–58.
3. Deenik AR, de Visser E, Louwerens JW, et al. Hallux valgus angle as a main predictor for correction of hallux valgus. BMC Musculoskelet Disord 2008;9:70.
4. Okuda R, Kinoshita M, Yasuda T, et al. Hallux valgus angle as a predictor of recurrence following proximal metatarsal osteotomy. J Orthop Sci 2011;16(6):760–4.
5. Okuda R, Kinoshita M, Yasuda T, et al. Postoperative incomplete reduction of the sesamoids as a risk factor for recurrence of hallux valgus. J Bone Joint Surg Am 2009;91(7):1637–45.
6. Paley D, Herzenberg J. Principles of Deformity Correction. Berlin Heidelberg (Germany): Springer-Verlag; 2002. p. 256–8.
7. Stienstra J, Lee A, Nakadate D. Large displacement distal chevron osteotomy for the correction of hallux valgus deformity. J Foot Ankle Surg 2002;41(4):213–20.
8. Dereymaeker G. Scarf osteotomy for correction of hallux valgus. Scarf technique and results as compared to distal chevron osteotomy. Foot Ankle Clin 2000;5(3): 513–24.
9. Wagner E, Ortiz C. Osteotomy considerations in hallux valgus treatment: improving the correction power. Foot Ankle Clin 2012;17:481–98.
10. Nyska M, Trnka HJ, Parks BG, et al. Proximal metatarsal osteotomies: a comparative geometric analysis conducted on sawbone models. Foot Ankle Int 2002;23: 938–45.
11. Mashima N, Yamamoto H, Tsuchiya H, et al. Correction of hallux valgus deformity using the center of rotation of angulation method. J Orthop Sci 2009;14:377–84.
12. Wagner E, Ortiz C, Keller A. Proximal oblique slide closing wedge metatarsal osteotomy with plate fixation for severe hallux valgus deformities. Tech Foot Ankle Surg 2007;6(4):270–4.
13. Kim Y, Kim J, Young K, et al. A new measure of tibial sesamoid position in hallux valgus in relation to the coronal rotation of the first metatarsal in CT scans. Foot Ankle Int 2015;36(8):944–52.
14. Yamaguchi S, Sasho T, Endo J, et al. Shape of the lateral edge of the first metatarsal head changes depending on the rotation and inclination of the first metatarsal: a study using digitally reconstructed radiographs. J Orthop Sci 2015;20:868–74.
15. Dayton P, Kauwe M, DiDomenico L, et al. Quantitative analysis of the degree of frontal rotation required to anatomically align the first metatarsal phalangeal joint during modified tarsal-metatarsal arthrodesis without capsular balancing. J Foot Ankle Surg 2016;55:220–5.
16. Wagner P, Ortiz C, Wagner E. Rotational osteotomy for hallux valgus. A new technique for primary and revision cases. Tech Foot Ankle Surg 2017;16(1):3–10.

Proximal Supination Osteotomy of the First Metatarsal for Hallux Valgus

Ryuzo Okuda, MD, PhD

KEYWORDS

- Hallux valgus • Surgical technique • Metatarsal osteotomy • Crescentic osteotomy
- Supination osteotomy • Pronation correction • Locking plate

KEY POINTS

- Varus and pronation of the first metatarsal are intimately related and seem to contribute to the development of hallux valgus.
- Postoperative pronation of the first metatarsal may cause risk factors, including a round lateral edge of the first metatarsal head (a positive round sign) and incomplete reduction of the sesamoids, for recurrence of hallux valgus.
- Proximal supination osteotomy of the first metatarsal facilitates correction of varus and pronation of the first metatarsal and achieves significant correction in moderate to severe hallux valgus deformities.
- Correcting pronation of the first metatarsal is effective in reducing postoperative recurrence of hallux valgus.

INTRODUCTION

Numerous investigators have reported the results of a proximal crescentic osteotomy combined with a distal soft tissue procedure and have recommended it for patients with moderate to severe hallux valgus.[1–14] However, postoperative recurrence of hallux valgus is a relatively common complication and is associated with unsatisfactory surgical outcomes.[1,7,11,15] Several investigators have reported that pronation of the first metatarsal is radiologically observed in patients with hallux valgus and suggested that pronation of the first metatarsal is intimately related and seems to contribute to the development of hallux valgus.[16–22] In addition, residual pronation of the first metatarsal after hallux valgus surgery may appear as a round lateral edge of the first metatarsal head (a positive round sign) and incomplete reduction of the sesamoids.[18,23] Based on these studies, some investigators recommended correction of pronation of the first metatarsal in hallux valgus surgery.[16–24] In a few

Department of Orthopaedic Surgery, Shimizu Hospital, 11-2 Yamadanakayoshimi-cho, Nishi-kyo-ku, Kyoto 615-8237, Japan
E-mail address: ryuokuda@car.ocn.ne.jp

Foot Ankle Clin N Am 23 (2018) 257–269
https://doi.org/10.1016/j.fcl.2018.01.006
1083-7515/18/© 2018 Elsevier Inc. All rights reserved.

foot.theclinics.com

recent studies, the pronation of the first metatarsal was corrected along with correction of the metatarsus primus varus to achieve better correction and to reduce the recurrence of hallux valgus; these investigators reported on the results of their surgical procedures.[13,23–26]

In 2007, the author devised a novel technique of a proximal supination osteotomy using Kirschner-wire fixation and performed this procedure for correction of moderate to severe hallux valgus. However, postoperative dorsiflexion deformity at the osteotomy site due to inadequate fixation was observed in a significant number of the patients.[13] Since 2012, the author has performed fixation of the osteotomy site with a locking X-plate. This article aims to describe the indication and surgical technique of a proximal supination osteotomy and to discuss the effect of pronation correction of the first metatarsal and stability of locking X-plate fixation at the osteotomy site in hallux valgus surgery.

INDICATIONS

The indications for a proximal supination osteotomy with a distal soft tissue procedure are (1) symptomatic moderate to severe hallux valgus deformity (a hallux valgus angle >25° and/or an intermetatarsal angle ≥12°) that has a round or intermediate-shaped lateral edge of the first metatarsal head on a preoperative dorsoplantar weight-bearing radiograph according to a measurement system[19] and (2) no response to conservative treatment, including modification of shoe wear, nonsteroidal antiinflammatory medication, or arch support. The shape of the lateral edge of the first metatarsal head, which consists of the articular surface and the lateral cortical surface of the metatarsal head on the dorsoplantar radiograph, is classified as one of 3 types, round (type R), angular (type A), or intermediate (type I) (**Fig. 1**). The round sign is positive when the shape of the lateral edge is classified as type R, and it is negative when the shape of the lateral edge is classified as type I or A.

Although there are no strict lower limits of a hallux valgus angle and an intermetatarsal angle in a proximal supination osteotomy, a mild hallux valgus deformity is mainly the indication for a distal metatarsal osteotomy.[27] The upper limits of the hallux valgus angle and an intermetatarsal angle, which can be corrected by a proximal supination osteotomy, are not identified. A proximal supination osteotomy can be performed in patients of all ages except patients with open physis.

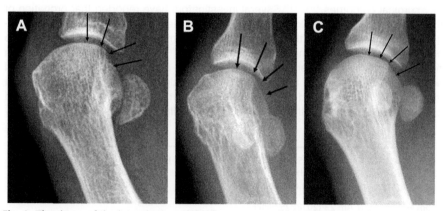

Fig. 1. The shape of the lateral edge of the first metatarsal head (*arrows*). (*A*) Angular: type A, (*B*) intermediate shape: type I, (*C*) round shape: type R.

CONTRAINDICATIONS

In the same way as a proximal metatarsal osteotomy, contraindications for a proximal supination osteotomy include the presence of severe osteoarthrosis and severe rheumatoid arthritis in the first metatarsophalangeal joint. The presence of severe soft tissue contracture in the first metatarsophalangeal joint and severe instability of the first tarsometatarsal (TMT) joint may be considered as contraindications.

Surgical Technique

The surgical technique consists of the release of the distal soft tissue, excision of the medial eminence, correction of metatarsus primus varus and pronation of the first metatarsal following a proximal crescentic osteotomy, internal fixation using the locking X-plate, and plication of the medial capsule.

Distal soft tissue procedure

Medial side of the first metatarsophalangeal joint A 3- to 4-cm curved skin incision convexing dorsally is made on the dorsomedial side of the first metatarsophalangeal joint. The adhesion between the subcutaneous tissue and the dorsal and medial parts of the capsule is carefully released. The dorsal digital nerve running on the dorsomedial aspect of the first metatarsophalangeal joint is exposed and is laterally retracted. When the dorsal cutaneous nerve adheres to the capsule and/or the expansion hood, neurolysis is performed. The abductor hallucis tendon is exposed at the medial side of the first metatarsophalangeal joint. The longitudinal capsulotomy is done at the dorsomedial aspect of the first metatarsophalangeal joint (**Fig. 2**A). The medial capsule and medial collateral ligament are then detached at the metatarsal head (**Fig. 2**B). The medial eminence of the metatarsal head is excised in line with the metatarsal shaft to preserve the distal articular surface of the metatarsal. The resection width of the medial eminence is around 2 mm.

Lateral side of the first metatarsophalangeal joint A 2-cm dorsal longitudinal skin incision is made between the first and second metatarsal heads. The lateral capsule and the adductor hallucis tendon are carefully exposed so as not to injure the deep peroneal nerve, which supplies the great toe and the second toe. The adductor hallucis tendon, including the transverse and oblique heads, is then dissected from its insertions at the base of the proximal phalanx and the lateral sesamoid (**Fig. 3**A). The transverse metatarsal ligament is released carefully so as not to injure the neurovascular bundle located directly under this ligament (**Fig. 3**B). A longitudinal

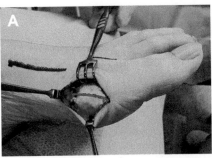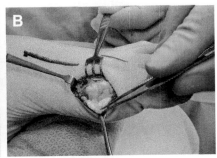

Fig. 2. (*A*) Longitudinal capsulotomy at the dorsomedial aspect of the first metatarsophalangeal joint (*red line*). (*B*) Detachment of the medial capsule and medial collateral ligament at the metatarsal head.

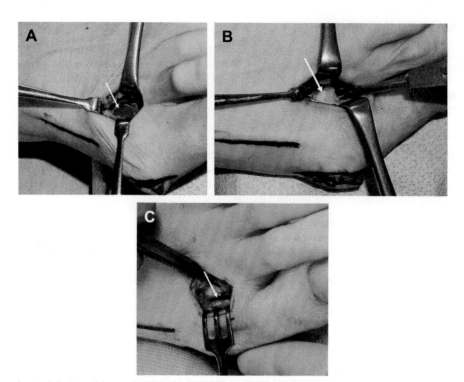

Fig. 3. (*A*) The adductor hallucis muscle and tendon (*arrow*). (*B*) The transverse metatarsal ligament (*arrow*) after dissection of the adductor hallucis tendon. (*C*) Longitudinal capsulotomy (*arrow*) at the dorsolateral aspect of the first metatarsophalangeal joint.

capsulotomy is made at the dorsolateral aspect of the first metatarsophalangeal joint so that the sesamoids are reduced under the metatarsal head as much as possible (**Fig. 3**C). Afterward, the operator confirms that the valgus deformity of the great toe can be manually corrected into 0° to 10° of varus (**Fig. 4**). If correction of the valgus

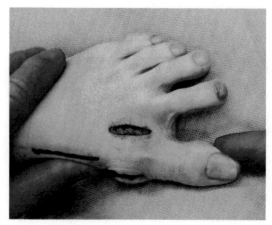

Fig. 4. Manual correction of a valgus deformity of the great toe showing 0° to 10° of varus position.

and pronation deformities in the great toe is not complete, additional release of the lateral capsule of the first metatarsophalangeal joint, including a part of the lateral collateral ligament, is required. However, excessive release of the lateral capsule should be avoided because it may lead to postoperative hallux varus.

Crescentic osteotomy

A 3- to 4-cm dorsomedial longitudinal skin incision is made over the first metatarsal base. The extensor halluces longus tendon is exposed so as not to injure the medial dorsal cutaneous nerve and the dorsal digital nerve. The longitudinal incision is made along the medial side of the extensor halluces longus tendon. The extensor halluces longus tendon is retracted laterally to expose the first metatarsal base. The periosteum of the first metatarsal base is longitudinally incised by a length of 3 to 4 cm, and the full circumferential release of the periosteum is performed. The first TMT joint is identified using the tip of an elevator. The osteotomy site, which is located 1.5 cm distal to the first TMT joint, is marked with a surgical marking pen. A crescentic osteotomy is performed with a curved saw blade. The osteotomy is curvilinear, and the concavity of the cut is directed proximally. The direction of the osteotomy is perpendicular to the soles of the feet on the coronal plane and is perpendicular to the long axis of the first metatarsal on the sagittal plane (**Fig. 5**).

Supination stress test of the great toe

After completion of a distal soft tissue procedure and a proximal crescentic osteotomy of the first metatarsal, supination stress of the great toe is performed to assess intraoperative correction of hallux valgus, metatarsus primus varus, the shape of the lateral edge of the first metatarsal, and the sesamoid position.[20] The maneuver of supination stress of the great toe is as follows: The plantar surface of the foot is placed on the image intensifier. The great toe is grasped; gentle axial traction is applied by pulling on the great toe, and then supination stress is manually applied to the great toe under dorsoplantar fluoroscopic view (**Fig. 6**A). Dorsoplantar fluoroscopic image of the foot is obtained under supination stress. When good corrections of a valgus deformity and metatarsus primus varus, reduction of the sesamoids, and a negative round sign of the lateral

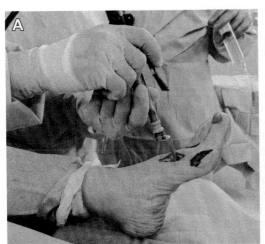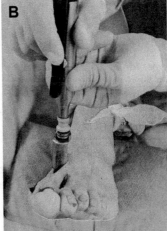

Fig. 5. (*A*) The direction of the osteotomy being perpendicular to the sole of the feet on the coronal plane and (*B*) perpendicular to the long axis of the first metatarsal on the sagittal plane.

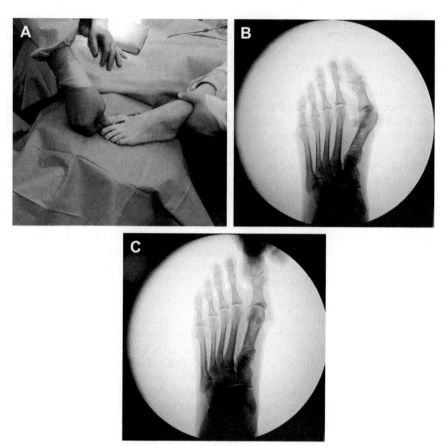

Fig. 6. Supination stress of the great toe. (*A*) Foot placement on the image intensifier. (*B*) Dorsoplantar fluoroscopic image under nonstress of the great toe. (*C*) Dorsoplantar fluoroscopic image under supination stress of the great toe.

edge of the first metatarsal head are observed, the release of the distal soft tissue and subperiosteum at the osteotomy site are considered to be adequate (**Fig. 6**B, C).

Correction at the osteotomy site

The proximal fragment is pushed medially with an elevator as much as possible; the distal fragment is moved laterally to achieve the parallel relationship between the first and second metatarsals, and then the distal fragment of the first metatarsal is manually supinated (**Fig. 7**). Temporary fixation with a 1.5-mm Kirschner wire is performed at the osteotomy site. And then the intermetatarsal angle and the shape of the lateral edge of the first metatarsal head on the dorsoplantar fluoroscopic view and the sagittal alignment of the osteotomy site on the lateral fluoroscopic view are checked. The author simulates the dorsoplantar weight-bearing view fluoroscopically as follows: the plantar surface of the foot is placed on the image intensifier with the ankle in 20° to 30°of plantarflexion and the metatarsophalangeal joint of the hallux in 10° to 20° of extension while patients are in the supine position. The lateral and medial sides of the forefoot and heel pad are simultaneously pushed manually toward the image intensifier. If the round or intermediate-shaped lateral edge of the first metatarsal head dose not changed to an angular lateral edge, further supination correction of

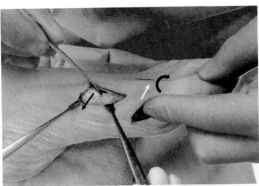

Fig. 7. Correction at the osteotomy site. The proximal fragment being pushed medially with an elevator (*black arrow*), and the distal fragment being moved laterally (*white arrow*) and supinated (*curved arrow*).

the proximal fragment is added so that the round or intermediate-shaped lateral edge of the metatarsal head on the dorsoplantar fluoroscopic view changes to an angular lateral edge. The author does not precisely measure the amount of supination to be achieved. The lateral fluoroscopic view is made as follows: the lateral side of the foot is placed on the image intensifier, and then the plantar surface of the foot is put on the plastic board with the ankle in 0° of plantarflexion. The lateral and medial sides of the forefoot sole and heel pad are placed simultaneously in contact with the plastic board. The direction of the fluoroscopic beam is parallel to the plastic board.

If the parallelism between the first and second metatarsals, the angular lateral edge (type A) on dorsoplantar fluoroscopic view, or good alignment of the first metatarsal on the lateral fluoroscopic view cannot be obtained, correction should be performed again. If good correction at the osteotomy site is obtained, another 1.5-mm Kirschner wire is inserted for temporary fixation at the osteotomy site.

Locking X-plate fixation

The variable angle (VA) locking X-plate has 4 holes and is available in extrasmall, small, medium, and large sizes (**Fig. 8**A). The appropriate locking X-plate size is selected using a template of each plate size, taking into account the relationship between the 4 screw holes of the locking X-plate and the proximal and distal fragments in order to achieve bicortical screw fixation in all screws. The author commonly uses the extra-small titanium VA locking X-plate, measuring 23.5 mm in length and 15.0 mm in width. When the bending of the locking X-plate is needed, the change of the screw direction due to the plate bending should be considered. After the VA locking X-plate is placed on the dorsal or dorsomedial aspect at the osteotomy site, the locking X-plate is fixed with 3 or 4 2.0-mm Kirschner wires, which is the same diameter of the drill hole for the head locking screw and can be inserted at −15° to +15° deviation from the center axis of the screw hole using the conical drill sleeve (**Fig. 8**B). After confirmation of the direction of the Kirschner wires, one Kirschner wire is removed and the head locking screw is inserted. The remaining 3 screws are then inserted in the same way. And then 2 Kirschner wires for temporary fixation at the osteotomy are removed.

Plication of the medial capsule

Two drill holes are made in the metatarsal neck and head using a 1.2-mm Kirschner wire. One is drilled at the dorsomedial side of the metatarsal head in the plantar to medial direction and the other at the dorsomedial side of the metatarsal neck in the

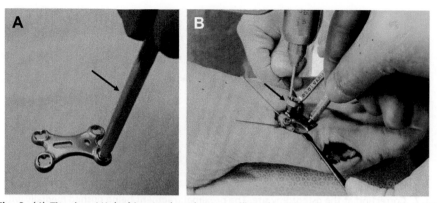

Fig. 8. (*A*) Titanium VA locking X-plate (extrasmall) with a plate holder (*arrow*). (*B*) A VA locking X-plate being temporally fixed with a 2.0-mm Kirschner wire using the conical drill sleeve (*arrow*) on the dorsal or dorsomedial aspect at the osteotomy site.

plantar direction. A 2-0 braided nonabsorbable suture is passed through each drill hole (**Fig. 9**). The medial part of the capsule, together with the abductor hallucis tendon, is proximally and dorsally pulled to correct the valgus and pronation deformities of the great toe and is fixed with 2 intraosseous sutures. And then the capsulorrhaphy is made with absorbable sutures.

Final fluoroscopic check

Intraoperative fluoroscopic dorsoplantar and lateral views of the foot are made to evaluate the hallux valgus angle (<15°), the intermetatarsal angle (<10°), the sesamoid position (<V according to Hardy classification), a round sign (negative), and sagittal alignment of the first metatarsal (no angulation at the osteotomy site) (**Fig. 10**).

Postoperative Treatment

A short-leg cast with rubber heel was continued for 2 weeks. Partial weight bearing was allowed 1 day after surgery. Two weeks after surgery, a short-leg plaster shell was applied and active and passive extension and flexion exercises of the first metatarsophalangeal joint was encouraged. Three weeks after surgery, patients were instructed to

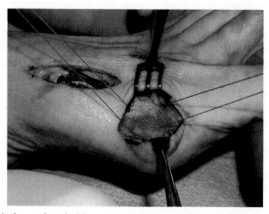

Fig. 9. A 2-0 braided nonabsorbable suture being passed through each drill hole.

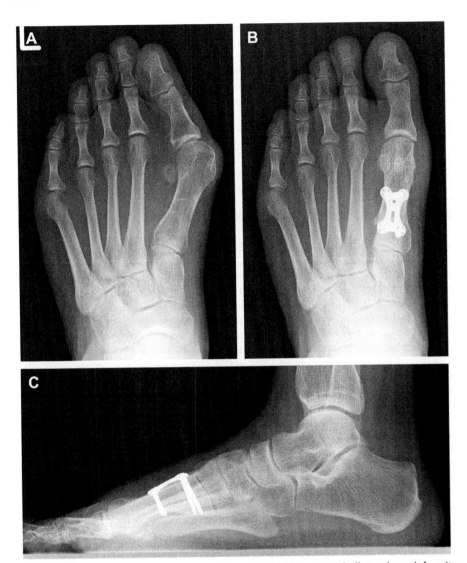

Fig. 10. (A) Preoperative dorsoplantar radiograph showing severe hallux valgus deformity with a grade VII position of the medial sesamoid and round lateral edge of the first metatarsal head (a positive round sign). (B) Dorsoplantar radiographs made 1 year postoperatively showing a hallux valgus angle of 10°, an intermetatarsal angle of 5°, a grade III position of the medial sesamoid, and angular lateral edge of the first metatarsal head (a negative round sign). (C) Lateral radiograph made 1 year postoperatively showing no dorsiflexion deformity of the first metatarsal.

wear street shoes with an arch support. Four weeks after surgery, full weight bearing was allowed. Patients could participate in sports activity 2 or 3 months after surgery.

Surgical Outcomes

Although a study on the results of a proximal supination osteotomy using a locking X-plate described here for correction of moderate and severe hallux valgus deformities is not yet reported, there are a few articles confirming the efficacy of pronation correction of the first metatarsal and/or reporting the results by different surgical procedures, including a proximal supination osteotomy using Kirschner wires,[13,23] the first TMT arthrodesis,[25,26] and a proximal rotational metatarsal osteotomy.[24] The author and colleagues[23] devised a new technique of proximal supination-abduction osteotomy and reviewed the short-term results of 12 adolescent feet with hallux valgus that underwent this procedure using Kirschner wires. They reported that the mean score by the Japanese Society for surgery of the foot standard rating system for hallux valgus improved significantly from 62.0 points preoperatively to 99.2 points postoperatively and the mean hallux valgus and intermetatarsal angles decreased significantly from 32.3° and 14.0° preoperatively to 12.2° and 6.2° postoperatively, respectively. Yasuda and colleagues[13] investigated the intermediate-term results of 83 adult feet that underwent a proximal supination osteotomy using Kirschner wires, which is the same as a proximal supination-abduction osteotomy described by the author and colleagues.[23] The investigators reported that the mean American Orthopedic Foot and Ankle Society hallux-metatarsophalangeal-interphalangeal (AOFAS) score improved significantly from 58.0 points preoperatively to 93.8 points postoperatively, and the mean hallux valgus and intermetatarsal angles decreased significantly from 38.6° and 18.0° preoperatively to 11.0° and 7.9° postoperatively, respectively. Dayton and colleagues[25] investigated the change in angular measurements in the evaluation of hallux valgus in 25 feet that underwent tarsal metatarsal corrective arthrodesis. They found that the mean hallux valgus and intermetatarsal angles decreased significantly from 30.3° and 14.9° preoperatively to 12.5° and 4.7° postoperatively, respectively, and recommended that rotational correction (pronation correction) of the first metatarsal is considered when correcting the hallux valgus deformity. Klemola and colleagues[26] investigated the 1-year radiological results of 84 feet that underwent the first TMT joint derotational (supination) arthrodesis without a distal soft tissue procedure and found that the mean hallux valgus and intermetatarsal angles decreased significantly from 30.5° and 13.2° preoperatively to 10.7° and 4.3° postoperatively, respectively, although any data regarding the clinical results were not presented in their study. They stated that the first TMT joint derotational (supination) arthrodesis showed notable correction of angle in hallux valgus. Wagner and colleagues[24] described a new technique of a proximal rotational metatarsal osteotomy and reported the short-term results of 6 feet that underwent this procedure. They found that the mean AOFAS score improved significantly from 55 points preoperatively to 85 points postoperatively and the mean hallux valgus and intermetatarsal angles decreased significantly from 35° and 16° preoperatively to 5° and 5° postoperatively, respectively.

Effect of Pronation Correction of the First Metatarsal

In hallux valgus surgery, recurrence is one of the most common complications and is associated with the deterioration of surgical outcomes.[1,7,11,28] Several investigators have reported a rate of postoperative recurrence of hallux valgus of 4% to 25% following proximal metatarsal osteotomy, although there were various definitions of recurrence among the articles.[1,3,5,9,11,13,29] The recurrence of hallux valgus may occur from various causes, including incomplete release of the soft tissue, insufficient plication of the medial capsule and the abductor hallucis tendon, insufficient correction of the metatarsus varus, increased distal metatarsal articular angle, a positive round sign at the lateral edge of the first metatarsal head, incomplete reduction of the sesamoids, and instability of the first TMT joint.[4,7,18,28,29]

A postoperative round sign of the first metatarsal head as a risk factor for recurrence of hallux valgus was significantly associated with pronation of the first metatarsal.[19,30,31] A positive round sign on a preoperative dorsoplantar radiograph may suggest that the first metatarsal is pronated. In such a case, pronation correction of the first metatarsal should be considered in hallux valgus surgery. In addition, residual pronation of the first metatarsal after hallux valgus surgery may be a possible component of incomplete reduction or lateral displacement of the sesamoids as a risk factor for recurrence.[29] Pronation of the first metatarsal simultaneously leads to pronation of the sesamoid articular surfaces of the first metatarsal head. Pronation of the sesamoid articular surfaces brings lateral displacement of these surfaces on the dorsoplantar plane compared with a normal foot. Even though the sesamoids are reduced to the articular surfaces when pronation of the first metatarsal is not corrected during surgery, lateral displacement of the sesamoids remains on the dorsoplantar plane. Therefore, correction of first metatarsal pronation in hallux valgus surgery should be considered to avoid a positive round sign and lateral displacement of the sesamoids.

Some surgical procedures in which pronation correction of the first metatarsal was done have been proposed for treating hallux valgus, and several investigators reported that pronation correction of the first metatarsal was effective for correction of the hallux valgus angle and intermetatarsal angle and reduction of the sesamoids.[13,23–26] The author and colleagues[23] and Yasuda and colleagues[13] found that a proximal supination osteotomy led to high rates of a negative round sign and complete reduction of the sesamoids postoperatively and described that these contributed to a low rate of recurrence of hallux valgus in their studies.

Stability of Locking X-Plate Fixation

Dorsiflexion of the distal fragment, which was caused by incorrect positioning of the distal fragment, inadequate fixation, or early postoperative weight bearing, is one of the common complications following a proximal crescentic osteotomy.[1,2,5,9,13,28,32] Mann and colleagues[1] found dorsiflexion deformity of the first metatarsal in 28% of patients who had a proximal crescentic osteotomy with screw fixation. Yasuda and colleagues[13] found dorsiflexion deformity in 23% of patients who had a proximal supination osteotomy with Kirschner-wire fixation and described that inadequate fixation seems to be the cause of postoperative dorsiflexion deformity. Rigid fixation is desirable to avoid dorsiflexion deformity, loss of correction, delayed union, or nonunion at the osteotomy site. Some investigators recommended plate fixation to address these concerns and improve stability instead of screw or Kirschner-wire fixation.[12,14,33,34] Chow and colleagues[12] reported on the long-term results of a proximal crescentic osteotomy using AO (Arbeitsgemeinschaft für Osteosynthesefragen) T-plate or L-plate and stated that good clinical and radiological results can be achieved. However, they did not report dorsiflexion deformity and loss of correction at the osteotomy site. Pauli and colleagues[14] investigated clinical outcomes and the fixation stability of a proximal crescentic osteotomy when using the small head locking X-plate and found satisfactory and reproducible results in terms of stability and bone healing. Ohbo and colleagues[35] investigated the stability of the VA locking X-plate fixation in a proximal supination osteotomy and stated that postoperative dorsiflexion deformity and loss of correction were not observed at the osteotomy site. The author thinks that the locking X-plate may provide a rigid fixation and lead to a low rate of dorsiflexion deformity and loss of correction in a proximal supination osteotomy, although further investigations are required.

REFERENCES

1. Mann RA, Rudicel S, Graves SC. Repair of hallux valgus with a distal soft-tissue procedure and proximal metatarsal osteotomy. A long-term follow-up. J Bone Joint Surg Am 1992;74:124–9.
2. Thordarson DB, Leventen EO. Hallux valgus correction with proximal metatarsal osteotomy: two-year follow-up. Foot Ankle 1992;13:321–6.
3. Dreeben S, Mann RA. Advanced hallux valgus deformity: long-term results utilizing the distal soft tissue procedure and proximal metatarsal osteotomy. Foot Ankle Int 1996;17:142–4.
4. Coughlin JM. Hallux valgus. J Bone Joint Surg Am 1996;78:932–66.
5. Easley ME, Kiebzak GM, Davis WH, et al. Prospective randomized comparison of proximal crescentic and proximal chevron osteotomies for correction of hallux valgus deformity. Foot Ankle Int 1996;17:307–16.
6. Markbreiter LA, Thompson FM. Proximal metatarsal osteotomy in hallux valgus correction: a comparison of crescentic and chevron procedures. Foot Ankle Int 1997;18:71–6.
7. Okuda R, Kinoshita M, Morikawa J, et al. Distal soft tissue procedure and proximal metatarsal osteotomy in hallux valgus. Clin Orthop Relat Res 2000;379:209–17.
8. Zettl R, Trnka HJ, Easley M, et al. Moderate to severe hallux valgus deformity: correction with proximal crescentic osteotomy and distal soft-tissue release. Arch Orthop Trauma Surg 2000;120:397–402.
9. Veri JP, Pirani SP, Clarige R. Crescentic proximal metatarsal osteotomy for moderate to severe hallux valgus: a mean 12.2 year follow-up study. Foot Ankle Int 2001;22:817–22.
10. Okuda R, Kinoshita M, Morikawa J, et al. Proximal metatarsal osteotomy. Relation between 1- to greater than 3-years results. Clin Orthop Relat Res 2005;435:191–6.
11. Coughlin MJ, Jones CP. Hallux valgus and first ray mobility. A prospective study. J Bone Joint Surg Am 2007;89:1887–98.
12. Chow FY, Lui TH, Kwok KW, et al. Plate fixation for crescentic metatarsal osteotomy in hallux valgus: an eight-year follow-up study. Foot Ankle Int 2008;29:29–33.
13. Yasuda T, Okuda R, Jotoku T, et al. Proximal supination osteotomy of the first metatarsal for hallux valgus. Foot Ankle Int 2015;36:696–704.
14. Pauli W, Koch A, Testa E, et al. Fixation of the proximal metatarsal crescentic osteotomy using a head locking X-plate. Foot Ankle Int 2016;37:218–26.
15. Sammarco GJ, Idusuyi OB. Complications after surgery of the hallux. Clin Orthop Relat Res 2001;391:58–71.
16. Mizuno S, Sima Y, Yamazaki K. Detorsion osteotomy of the first metatarsal bone in hallux valgus. J Jpn Orthop Assoc 1956;30:813–9.
17. Eustace S, Obyrne J, Stack J, et al. Radiographic features that enable the assessment of first metatarsal rotation: the role of pronation in hallux valgus. Skeletal Radiol 1993;22:153–6.
18. Saltzman CL, Brandser EA, Anderson CM, et al. Coronal plane rotation of the first metatarsal. Foot Ankle Int 1996;17:157–61.
19. Okuda R, Kinoshita M, Toshito Y, et al. The shape of the lateral edge of the first metatarsal head as a risk factor for recurrence of hallux valgus. J Bone Joint Surg Am 2007;89:2163–72.
20. Okuda R, Yasuda T, Jotoku T, et al. Supination stress of the great toe for assessing intraoperative correction of hallux valgus. J Orthop Sci 2012;17:129–35.

21. Mortier JP, Bernard JL, Maestro M. Axial rotation of the first metatarsal head in a normal population and hallux valgus patients. Orthop Traumatol Surg Res 2012; 98:677–83.
22. Dayton P, Feilmeier M, Hirschi J, et al. Observed changes in radiographic measurements of the first ray after frontal plane rotation of the first metatarsal in a cadaveric foot model. J Foot Ankle Surg 2014;53:274–8.
23. Okuda R, Yasuda T, Jotoku T, et al. Proximal abduction–supination osteotomy of the first metatarsal for adolescent hallux valgus: a preliminary report. J Orthop Sci 2013;18:129–35.
24. Wagner P, Ortiz C, Wagner E, et al. Rotational osteotomy for hallux valgus. A new technique for primary and revision cases. Tech Foot Ankle Surg 2017;16:3–10.
25. Dayton P, Feilmeier M, Kauwe M, et al. Relationship of frontal plane rotation of first metatarsal to proximal articular set angle and hallux alignment in patients undergoing tarsometatarsal arthrodesis for hallux abducto valgus: a case series and critical review of the literature. J Foot Ankle Surg 2013;52:348–54.
26. Klemola T, Leppilahti J, Kalinainen S, et al. First tarsometatarsal joint derotational arthrodesis: a new operative technique for flexible hallux valgus without touching the first metatarsophalangeal joint. J Foot Ankle Surg 2014;53:22–8.
27. Pinney SJ, Song KR, Chou LB. Surgical treatment of mild hallux valgus deformity: the state of practice among academic foot and ankle surgeons. Foot Ankle Int 2006;27:970–3.
28. Okuda R, Kinoshita M, Yasuda T, et al. Postoperative incomplete reduction of the sesamoids as a risk factor for the recurrence of hallux valgus. J Bone Joint Surg Am 2009;91:1637–45.
29. Shurnas PS, Watson TS, Crislip TW. Proximal first metatarsal opening wedge osteotomy with a low profile plate. Foot Ankle Int 2009;30:865–72.
30. Iyer S, Demetracopoulos CA, Sofka CM, et al. High rate of recurrence following proximal medial opening wedge osteotomy for correction of moderate hallux valgus. Foot Ankle Int 2015;36:756–63.
31. Yamaguchi S, Sasho T, Endo J, et al. Shape of the lateral edge of the first metatarsal head changes depending on the rotation and inclination of the first metatarsal: a study using digitally reconstructed radiographs. J Orthop Sci 2015;20: 868–74.
32. Dayton P, Kauwe M, DiDomenico L, et al. Quantitative analysis of the degree of frontal rotation required to anatomically align the first metatarsal phalangeal joint during modified tarsal-metatarsal arthrodesis without capsular balancing. J Foot Ankle Surg 2016;55:220–5.
33. Brodsky JW, Beischer AD, Robinson AHN, et al. Surgery for hallux valgus with proximal crescentic osteotomy causes variable postoperative pressure patterns. Clin Orthop Relat Res 2006;443:280–6.
34. Rosenberg GA, Donley BG. Plate augmentation of screw fixation of proximal crescentic osteotomy of the first metatarsal. Foot Ankle Int 2003;24:570–1.
35. Ohbo T, Okuda R, Fukunishi K, et al. Proximal supination osteotomy using locking plate for correction of hallux valgus. Cent Japan J Orthop Traumatol (in Japanese) 2015;58:745–6.

Hallux Valgus Deformity and Treatment

A Three-Dimensional Approach

Jesse Forbes Doty, MD[a], Wallace Taylor Harris, MD[b],*

KEYWORDS

- First metatarsocuneiform joint • Hypermobility • Hallux valgus • First ray
- Intermetatarsal angle • Hallux valgus angle

KEY POINTS

- Normal mobility of the first ray consists of an axis from dorsal-medial to plantar-lateral.
- Because of the complexity of the three-dimensional anatomy of the first metatarsocuneiform (MTC) joint, it is imperative that radiographs are standardized and consistent during evaluation.
- Hypermobility of the first ray, in association with hallux valgus, is not an absolute indication for first MTC arthrodesis.

INTRODUCTION

Motion and spatial orientation of the first metatarsocuneiform (MTC) joint has been shown to have significant clinical implications. The planes of motion make the two major axes of the first MTC joint move in a dorsal-medial to plantar-lateral direction. The contribution of each, especially mobility via the sagittal plane, in the development of hallux valgus deformities is at the center of much debate (**Fig. 1**).

Morton[1-3] was the first to suggest first MTC hypermobility contributed to multiple conditions of the foot and ankle. He made no connection with the development of hallux valgus at that time. There are 2 major planes of motion involved with hallux valgus deformity. To patients, the deformity in the transverse plane is most glaring and what they attribute their bunion to originate from. To the clinician, it is a much more complicated matter, as this relationship between the deformity in the

Disclosure Statement: The authors have nothing to disclose.
[a] UT Erlanger Orthopaedics, University of Tennessee College of Medicine, 979 East Third Street C225, Chattanooga, TN 37405, USA; [b] UT Erlange Orthopaedics, University of Tennessee College of Medicine, Chattanooga, TN 37405, USA
* Corresponding author. 201 Cherokee Boulevard, Apartment 407, Chattanooga, TN 37405.
E-mail address: wtharri@gmail.com

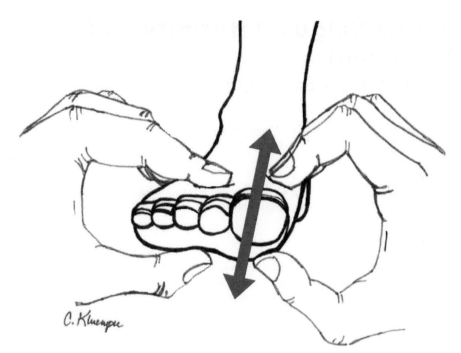

Fig. 1. First ray axis of motion. The first ray axis moves from dorsal-medial to plantar-lateral. *Courtesy of* Chase Kluemper, MD, University of Tennessee Orthopedic Surgery, Chattanooga, TN.

transverse plane and motion in the sagittal plane is more involved. It has been paralleled by some investigators to the philosophic debate of which came first, the chicken or the egg?

There is a sparse amount of objective literature supporting either camp of thought, though recent evidence has provided some clarity.[4,5] Many think it is the transverse plane deformity involving hallux valgus with the sagittal plane hypermobility resulting secondarily and not acting as the primary deforming force.[6-11] Others claim those patients with higher motion in the sagittal plane are predisposed to the development of transverse plane malalignment and hallux valgus deformity.[12-17] Further ambiguity arises in the lack of uniformity from an imaging and radiographic standpoint.[5] To have a fair debate, the terms must be defined and they must be as objective as possible. Because of the complexity of the three-dimensional anatomy of the first MTC joint, slight changes in position can cause significant changes in radiographic measurements and manual examination findings used for clinical evaluation.[5,18]

Questions to Be Answered

The following are pertinent questions related to first ray hypermobility and its relationship to hallux valgus:

Is first ray hypermobility a pathologic entity?

Morton[1-3] and Lapidus[19] theorized that hypermobility of the first ray originated from the first MTC joint and that stabilizing this would normalize mobility and correct the hallux valgus deformity. This theory was later supported by Lee and Young,[15] Klaue and colleagues,[14] and Faber and colleagues[20] who associated increased sagittal plane mobility with hallux valgus.

How should mobility of the first ray be objectively measured, and what is the threshold for hypermobile versus nonhypermobile?

Morton was the first to describe proper manual examination of first ray hypermobility.[1–3,11]

The examination is performed with the ankle in neutral dorsiflexion. The examiner places one hand on the lateral aspect of the forefoot at the metatarsal heads with the other hand grasping the first ray. The first metatarsal is then mobilized by the examiner in a dorsal-plantar direction. The amount of motion is estimated and graded. Grading of the mobility is measured with the descriptors mild, moderate, substantial mobility, and hypermobile.

Morton's manual physical examination was then tested for reliability.[21] Glasoe and colleagues[21] had both physicians and physical therapists measure using the terms of hypermobility from Morton's original work. Intrarater and interrater reliability were analyzed separately. Intrarater reliability showed agreement with little consistency in interrater reliability. This finding emphasized that although a single practitioner could show consistency in measuring the same foot for multiple examinations, there is little clinical objectivity to comparing magnitudes between examiners. This study documented a need for increased reliability in measurements of first ray mobility.

The Klaue device sought to provide clarity. The device functions as an ankle-foot-orthosis with an external caliper providing plantar to dorsal forces. Using the device, Klaue and colleagues[14] showed on average, patients without hallux valgus deformity had 5 mm of motion while those with hallux valgus deformity had 8 mm. The device was further validated by Jones and colleagues[10] using cadavers. A similar device was created by Glasoe and colleagues[22] with the main difference being the origin of the force produced for the plantar to dorsal movements, man versus machine. Although both devices greatly increased the ability to objectively measure mobility of the first ray, neither device specifically isolates motion to the first MTC joint. Along with providing a more reliable way to measure the mobility of the first ray, these studies served to set parameters for normal versus abnormal motion.

In addition to the poor inter-reliability found by Glasoe and colleagues[21] regarding Morton's manual examination, Grebing and Coughlin[23] evaluated the effect of ankle position on the examination of first ray mobility. They studied 4 groups in total:

1. Control group/healthy subjects
2. Moderate to severe hallux valgus deformity
3. Patients with prior MTP arthrodesis for hallux valgus deformity with all nonunions excluded
4. Patients who had previously undergone plantar fasciectomy

Using the Klaue device for measurements, they found all patients showed decreased first ray mobility in the dorsiflexed position compared with neutral and increased mobility in the plantar-flexed position except for the plantar fasciectomy group. Along with stating the recommendations for manual examination of the first ray, the investigators emphasized correct and consistent positioning of the ankle when evaluating mobility of the first ray. The suggestion is also made that flexion of the knee during examination can relieve tension at the plantar aponeurosis allowing mobility of the first ray to be better isolated.

Given the ability to quantify hypermobility of the first ray, what are its clinical implications in the development of hallux valgus deformities and its relationship to the first metatarsocuneiform joint?

Understanding the anatomic, biomechanical, and radiographic characteristics of the first MTC joint is essential to properly understand whether mobility is a primary force or secondary result of hallux valgus deformity and other foot pathology.

RELEVANT ANATOMY OF THE FIRST METATARSOCUNEIFORM JOINT
First Metatarsocuneiform Joint Anatomy

The first ray consists of the 3 major components: the great toe phalanges, the first metatarsal, and the medial cuneiform. In conjunction with the first ray, the naviculocuneiform and talonavicular joints combine to complete the medial column. The mean height of the MTC joint from dorsal to plantar is 28.3 mm with the average width from medial to lateral being 13.1 mm.[5] This 2:1 ratio has been validated by multiple studies.[24] There are 2 main facets of the first MTC joint: dorsal and plantar. Variability exists between the facets, as 59% show a continuous cartilaginous surface, 38% show a bilobed cartilaginous surface, and 3% demonstrate a complete separation of the articular surfaces.[5] Fifteen percent of specimens show an intermetatarsal facet between the first and second metatarsals. Other studies have reported a higher incidence of intermetatarsal facets (29%) and correlated this with increased amounts of medial inclination.[25,26] Wanivenhaus and Pretterklieber[24] had a more equivalent prevalence of continuous and bilobed facets. In regard to predicting hallux valgus deformities, having continuous facets seems to increase the likelihood of having a higher 1 to 2 intermetatarsal angle. There was no correlation between magnitude of the hallux valgus angle (HVA) and the presence of continuous facets.[5] In comparison, the dorsal facet was almost always (95%) convex in nature, whereas the plantar facet was seen to be more commonly flat (77%). Contour differences between the dorsal and plantar facets did not correlate with hypermobility or the presence of hallux valgus deformity.[5]

In relation to the second MTC joint, the first MTC joint is typically found more distally along the long axis of the foot as it articulates with the base of the first metatarsal. The joint convexity is on the medial cuneiform with the base of the first metatarsal remaining concave. Medial deviation is the most commonly described orientation.[5] This medial deviation can be highly variable based on true patient anatomy as well as radiographic positioning and measurement parameters.

Normal Mobility of the First Ray

Movement in the dorsal and plantar direction in the sagittal plane is most significant. Approximately 10% of specimens lack the ability to reach significant abduction/adduction in the transverse plane.[24] In comparison with the naviculocuneiform and talonavicular joints, the first MTC joint contributes most of both sagittal and transverse plane movement for the first ray; it has a larger share of the transverse plane comparatively[20]: specifically, 82% for the transverse/medial mobility and 57% for the dorsal/sagittal motion.

Soft Tissue Contributions Relative to the First Metatarsocuneiform Joint
Tibialis anterior

In both the sagittal and transverse planes, the tibialis anterior muscle does not play a significant role in mobility at the first MTC joint. From a pure functionality standpoint, it acts to dorsiflex the first ray through its vector of pull.[20]

Peroneus longus

The peroneus longus muscle plays a significant role in the stability at the first MTC joint in both the sagittal and transverse planes.[20,27] It plays a larger role in dorsal stability in the sagittal plane compared with medial deviation in the transverse plan. Unlike Bohne and colleagues,[27] Faber and colleagues[20] did not find a statistically significant role in medial stability. From a functionality standpoint, the peroneus longus muscle acts as a strong plantar flexor of the first ray, which would counteract dorsal displacement.

Flexor hallucis longus

Similar to the peroneus longus muscle, the flexor hallucis muscle provides significant contribution seen with dorsal and medial stability with a larger relative contribution in the sagittal plane.[20] In the sagittal plane, the flexor hallucis longus (FHL) acts as a primary plantar flexor, thus, counteracting dorsal displacement. In the transverse plane, the FHL may further perpetuate the hallux valgus deformity and has been shown to have an increasing effect on medial deviation of the first metatarsal.[28] Faber and colleagues[20] found similar results in both the sagittal and transverse planes.

RADIOGRAPHIC CHARACTERISTICS

Recent quantitative, objective studies have made advances in delineating the contributions of the first MTC to hallux valgus deformities with much of this focused on radiographic measurements. Anteroposterior (AP), modified 10° to 20° AP, and lateral radiographs serve as the standard images when evaluating the first MTC joint.[5] With regard to hallux valgus deformities, little data exist to warrant further imaging workup with computed tomography or MRI to specifically evaluate the MTC joint. Depending on the orientation of the joint on AP and lateral radiographs, the accuracy of measurements can be altered and make results of various studies hard to compare.

In regard to hallux valgus deformity and its relationship with the first MTC joint, radiographic angles of greatest importance are the HVA, the 1 to 2 intermetatarsal angle (IMA), and the medial and lateral inclination angles of the first MTC joint. The HVA is formed by 2 tangential lines formed down the longitudinal axis of the first metatarsal and the first proximal phalanx on AP weight-bearing radiographs. Normal angulation is defined as less than 15° with mild, moderate, and severe deformities accordingly at 15° to 20°, 20° to 40°, and greater than 40°.[7] The IMA is formed by 2 tangential lines formed down the longitudinal axis of the first and second metatarsals on AP weight-bearing radiographs. Normal angulation is less than 9° with mild, moderate, and severe deformity defined as less than 11°, 11° to 16°, and greater than 16°.[7] Medial inclination angle is measured on AP radiographs as the angle between the distal articular surface of the cuneiform relative to the transverse tarsal line.[5] Lateral inclination angle is measured on lateral radiographs as the angle formed between a line perpendicular to the plantar aspect of the foot and one tangential with the first MTC joint.[5] Furthermore, the lateral inclination angle can be specific to both the dorsal and plantar facets of the first cuneiform.

These angles are greatly affected by the angle of the radiographic beam. In addition to the appropriate beam angle for both medial and lateral inclination, it is important to understand the percentage of representation for the plantar versus dorsal facet with regard to the image produced. The dorsal facet tends to be more vertically oriented compared with the plantar facet. Depending on the angulation of the radiographic beam, varying amounts of each facet would be shown in profile on AP films. By increasing the radiographic beam's angulation, a greater proportion of the plantar facet is seen. This image may reveal the flatter plantar facet compared with the more convex/contoured dorsal facet and can change an examiner's interpretation of the first MTC architecture.[5] Brage and colleagues[18] compared AP radiographs at 10° and 20° and saw on average a 7.2° increase in medial inclination. Doty and colleagues[5] found similar results comparing the medial inclination on equivalent radiographs at a 13.2° increase for 10° versus 20° AP radiographs.

Morton[2] discussed cortical thickening of the second metatarsal on AP radiographs as a key premise to his theory about first ray instability. He proposed that increased motion of the first ray would lead to greater force delivered through the second metatarsal leading to hypertrophic changes. This was used when deciding treatment options for hallux valgus deformity, whether first MTC arthrodesis would be beneficial. This idea was later disputed by Grebing and Coughlin[29] who compared second metatarsal cortical thickness with hallux valgus, hallux rigidus, and interdigital neuromas and found no correlation. The radiographic evaluation of the first MTC joint is complex and requires an in-depth understanding of the three-dimensional anatomy.

Clinical Relevance

Our understanding is ever evolving in the interplay between first ray hypermobility, hallux valgus deformity, and the first MTC joint. Studies have linked hallux valgus deformity to first ray hypermobility, specifically targeting the first MTC joint, with most efforts focusing on mobility in the sagittal plate. Many surgeons think that by correcting excess motion at the first MTC joint via arthrodesis, this would then normalize hypermobility of the first ray and would address the primary cause of the hallux valgus deformity.[12,13,16,19,24,30] Hallux valgus deformities with concomitant first ray hypermobility, whether measured via clinical examination or objectively, would best be treated with first MTC joint arthrodesis. Recent literature has focused efforts to objectively measure first ray hypermobility in an attempt to quantify the contributing factors. There is some disagreement with prior indications for first MTC arthrodesis. Studies have shown realignment procedures at the first metatarsophalangeal joint effect vectors of soft tissue support, which serve to stabilize the medial column without arthrodesis of the MTC joint.[29] First ray hypermobility or lack thereof is multifactorial and may not be as simple as previously described with regard to inherent skeletal instability.[6–11,31]

Klaue and colleagues[14] studied this objectively using their device that has since been validated. They compared 3 groups of patients:

1. Asymptomatic, normal population being seen in clinic for other complaints
2. Patients with symptomatic, hallux valgus deformity with HVA greater than 20°
3. Patients with foot deformities other than hallux valgus

The patients with hallux valgus deformity had increased passive elevation of the first ray. The investigators suggested this links hypermobility of the first ray to hallux valgus deformity, as patients without hallux valgus deformity averaged 5 mm of movement, whereas those with hallux valgus were seen to have 8 mm. Although they address some of the lack of objectivity with this link by using the Klaue device, it still fails to pinpoint this movement to the first MTC joint, as this is only one component of the first ray.

Lee and Young[15] attempted to further validate the link to hallux valgus deformity though they use a different threshold for hypermobile versus nonhypermobile. They defined hypermobility of the first ray by greater than 14° which correlates with greater than the 95th percentile in normal subjects without hallux valgus. The authors used a method for calculating mobility through a combination of radiographs and physical examination measurements. The results revealed 12.9 versus 10.3° of motion in the hallux valgus group compared with healthy subjects. Without the use of an established device for measurements, the methods of measuring mobility of the first ray was less objective.

Clinical trials have established first MTC arthrodesis as an appropriate treatment option for hallux valgus deformity with first ray hypermobility.[12,17] Myerson and colleagues[16] evaluated 67 cases of first MTC arthrodesis. The patients were followed clinically for an average of 28 months with preoperative and postoperative radiographs. The average HVA correction was 35° to 13° postoperatively, with the IMA correction from 14° to 6°. Eight-five percent of patients had normal first ray motion postoperatively via clinical examination. There was no objective measurement of first ray motion. The investigators concluded that first MTC arthrodesis was a reliable treatment option for hallux valgus deformity with metatarsus primus varus, and 77% of patients had total relief. Ellington and colleagues[13] later reported on the Lapidus procedure for the treatment of recurrent hallux valgus deformity with excellent radiographic correction and low nonunion rates.

Sangeorzan and Hansen[17] reported on the modified Lapidus procedure in 33 patients with 40 total operatively treated feet. Thirty-three of the feet were defined as having a hypermobile first ray by lacking an end point with dorsal stress on physical examination. The average preoperative IMA was 14°, with an average HVA of 26°. Postoperatively, the IMA corrected to 6° with the HVA decreasing to 11°. Five of the 40 operatively treated feet required reoperation (13%). Reasons for repeat operation included hallux varus deformity, recurrent hallux valgus deformity, nonunion, and transfer metatarsalgia. The investigators concluded that the modified Lapidus procedure is an acceptable treatment option but, secondary to the technical difficulty, should be reserved for severe IMAs, recurrent deformities failing prior treatments, and patients with hypermobility of the first ray. The investigators did not characterize postoperative first ray mobility.

Some publications have objectively measured first ray hypermobility and attempted to characterize whether correcting the first MTC joint is necessary to successfully treat hallux valgus deformity. Coughlin and colleagues[6] evaluated arthrodesis at the first MTP joint and its effects on first ray hypermobility. In these patients, the average corrections of the HVA and IMA were 21° and 6°, respectively. The average postoperative dorsiflexion angle was 22° at the MTP joint. At an average of 8 years postoperatively, 16 patients (21 feet) had on average 3.9 mm of dorsiflexion of the first ray. Although there were no preoperative measurements to compare with, this suggested that any hypermobility present preoperatively was corrected without fusion at the first MTC joint. There were no patients with documented ligamentous laxity using the Beighton 9-point examination.

First metatarsophalangeal arthrodesis has been well established as a valid treatment option for hallux valgus deformity. Cronin and colleagues[32] showed similar correction of IMA of 8.2° in cases of severe hallux valgus after treatment with MTP fusion. The mean preoperative HVA in their patients was 46.5°. Correction of the IMA is seen immediately postoperatively but improved from 6 weeks to the final follow-up visit. This correction could be secondary to a lack of immediate weight-bearing radiographs taken postoperatively as well as continued improvement in the IMA. Lastly, Mann and Katcherian[30] found similar IMA corrections as did Humbert, Coughlin, and Cronin with overall correction of 4.4°. Mann and Katcherian included hallux rigidus, hallux varus, and those with prior osteotomies with hallux valgus, which all would tend to have lower IMAs preoperatively. In addition, the investigators deemed a proximal osteotomy unnecessary to correct the IMA as MTP arthrodesis was sufficient.

Grimes and Coughlin[33] evaluated first MTP fusion for the treatment of recurrent hallux valgus deformity. They showed good results with only 2 of 29 patients demonstrating first ray hypermobility at 8 years postoperatively as measured with the Klaue device. Of these 2 patients, both demonstrated ligamentous laxity and maintained good satisfaction scores and correction on radiographs until final follow-up. Kim and colleagues[11] evaluated the effects of a proximal metatarsal chevron osteotomy with distal soft tissue procedure in hallux valgus deformity corrections in patients with first ray hypermobility. They measured the dorsiflexion mobility of the first ray preoperatively and 1 year postoperatively using the Klaue device. The mean preoperative dorsiflexion was 6.8 mm with the mean postoperative mobility at 1 year being 3.2 mm. They had no recurrence of deformity. This finding was statistically significant, and the investigators concluded that performing this combination of osteotomy and soft tissue procedures was a valid treatment option for patients with symptomatic hallux valgus with concomitant first ray hypermobility. Their findings suggest that hypermobility of the first ray is multifactorial and that it was unnecessary to violate the first MTC joint to achieve decreased mobility and correction of deformity.

Coughlin and Shurnas[9] studied first ray hypermobility after the distal soft tissue procedure and proximal metatarsal osteotomy for the treatment of hallux valgus in men. They used the Klaue device to measure first ray mobility postoperatively, as the device was not available preoperatively. They compared the operative first ray mobility with the nonoperative side in the same patient. The authors found no statistically significant difference between the operative and nonoperative sides, as the operative side had a mean mobility of 4.9 mm compared with 5.6 mm on the normal side. In addition, there was no association between hallux valgus deformity and metatarsus adductus, pes planus, or heel cord tightness.

Coughlin and Jones[7] performed a prospective study on distal soft tissue procedure and proximal metatarsal osteotomy (DSTP-PMO) on first ray hypermobility. The average follow-up was 27 months with a total of 127 feet evaluated both preoperatively and postoperatively with the Klaue device. They found a reduction from 7.2 mm to 4.5 mm after DSTP-PMO was performed. Although correction of the coronal deformity involving the first MTC joint is necessary, correcting the hallux valgus deformity and decreasing sagittal plane motion without violating the MTC joint led the investigators to think the sagittal plane hypermobility was a secondary result and not the primary cause of hallux valgus deformity.

Faber and colleagues[31] performed a prospective study comparing the distal osteotomy of the first metatarsal (Hohmann procedure) with first tarsometatarsal joint fusion and soft tissue procedure of the first metatarsophalangeal joint (the Lapidus procedure) in patients with hallux valgus deformity. They looked at 101 feet from 87 patients. They excluded patients treated with a first MTP arthrodesis or inflammatory arthropathies and any patients with prior surgeries to the involved medial column. Mobility was measured by manual examination with displacement greater than 8 to 10 mm classified as hypermobility. Seventy-one percent of the patients treated with the Lapidus procedure were hypermobile preoperatively, whereas 64% from the Hohmann group were classified as hypermobile. There was no difference in outcomes between the two treatment arms or between those patients labeled hypermobile and nonhypermobile. Similar results were seen with improvements in pain scores and patient satisfaction between the two groups. The investigators concluded that hallux valgus in the presence of hypermobility of the first ray may be successfully treated without first MTC arthrodesis.

Coughlin and colleagues[8] performed a cadaveric study in order to measure the immediate effects of DSTP-PMO on sagittal plane mobility. The investigators recorded a decrease in sagittal plane motion in their cadaveric specimens from 11.0 mm to 5.2 mm after DSTP-PMO. They noted a trend toward increasing first ray mobility in the sagittal plane with a magnitude of hallux valgus deformity based on IMA and HVA with normal restoration possible without violating the first MTC joint.

SUMMARY

Procedures involving first MTC fusion are technically demanding, and some investigators suggest fusion should be reserved for cases with MTC arthritis or more severe hallux valgus deformity cases in which the IMA cannot be improved by a metatarsal shaft osteotomy. Nonunion, hardware removal and failure, metatarsalgia, and bone grafting are mentioned as factors leading to greater patient morbidity. The cause and effect between hallux valgus and first ray hypermobility continues to be debated. Understanding the anatomic and radiographic examination of the first MTC joint is critical to choosing an appropriate treatment algorithm for the surgical management of hallux valgus deformity. Some studies suggest hypermobility can be corrected without fusing the first MTC joint. Many investigators think hypermobility arises secondarily from malalignment of the soft tissue constraints as the hallux valgus deformity progresses. Other investigators think hypermobility is a primary cause of the hallux valgus deformity and have reported good results with surgical correction including a first TMT arthrodesis.

REFERENCES

1. Morton D. Hypermobility of the first metatarsal bone: the interlinking factor between metatarsalgia and longitudinal arch strains. J Bone Joint Surg 1928;10: 187–96.
2. Morton D. Significant characteristics of the Neanderthal foot. Nat Hist 1926;26: 310–4.
3. Morton D. The human foot. New York: Columbia University Press; 1935.
4. Doty JF, Coughlin MJ. Hallux valgus and hypermobility of the first ray: facts and fiction. Int Orthop 2013;37(9):1655–60.
5. Doty JF, Coughlin MJ, Hirose C, et al. First metatarsocuneiform joint mobility. Foot Ankle Int 2014;35(5):504–11.
6. Coughlin MJ, Grebing BR, Jones CP. Arthrodesis of the first metatarsophalangeal joint for idiopathic hallux valgus: intermediate results. Foot Ankle Int 2005;26(10): 783–92.
7. Coughlin J, Jones CP. Hallux valgus and first ray mobility. A prospective study. J Bone Joint Surg Am 2007;89(9):1887–98.
8. Coughlin MJ, Jones CP, Viladot R, et al. Hallux valgus and first ray mobility: a cadaveric study. Foot Ankle Int 2004;25(8):537–44.
9. Coughlin MJ, Shurnas PS. Hallux valgus in men part II: first ray mobility after bunionectomy and factors associated with hallux valgus deformity. Foot Ankle Int 2003;24(1):73–8.
10. Jones CP, Coughlin MJ, Pierce-Villadot R, et al. The validity and reliability of the Klaue device. Foot Ankle Int 2005;26(11):951–6.
11. Kim J-Y, Park JS, Hwang SK, et al. Mobility changes of the first ray after hallux valgus surgery: clinical results after proximal metatarsal chevron osteotomy and distal soft tissue procedure. Foot Ankle Int 2008;29(5):468–72.
12. Bednarz PA, Manoli A. Modified Lapidus procedure for the treatment of hypermobile hallux valgus. Foot Ankle Int 2000;21(10):816–21.
13. Ellington JK, Myerson MS, Coetzee JC, et al. The use of the Lapidus procedure for recurrent hallux valgus. Foot Ankle Int 2011;32(7):674–80.
14. Klaue K, Hansen ST, Masquelet AC. Clinical, quantitative assessment of first tarsometatarsal mobility in the sagittal plane and its relation to hallux valgus deformity. Foot Ankle Int 1994;15(1):9–13.

15. Lee KT, Young K. Measurement of first-ray mobility in normal vs. hallux valgus patients. Foot Ankle Int 2001;22(12):960–4.
16. Myerson M, Allon S, Mcgarvey W. Metatarsocuneiform arthrodesis for management of hallux valgus and metatarsus primus varus. Foot Ankle 1992;13(3): 107–15.
17. Sangeorzan BJ, Hansen ST. Modified Lapidus procedure for hallux valgus. Foot Ankle 1989;9(6):262–6.
18. Brage ME, Holmes JR, Sangeorzan BJ. The influence of X-Ray orientation on the first metatarsocuneiform joint angle. Foot Ankle Int 1994;15(9):495–7.
19. Lapidus PW. The author's bunion operation from 1931 to 1959. Clin Orthop 1960; 16:119–35.
20. Faber FW, Kleinrensink G-J, Verhoog MW, et al. Mobility of the first tarsometatarsal joint in relation to hallux valgus deformity: anatomical and biomechanical aspects. Foot Ankle Int 1999;20(10):651–6.
21. Glasoe WM, Allen MK, Saltzman CL, et al. Comparison of two methods used to assess first-ray mobility. Foot Ankle Int 2002;23(3):248–52.
22. Glasoe WM, Yack H, Saltzman CL. Measuring first ray mobility with a new device. Arch Phys Med Rehabil 1999;80(1):122–4.
23. Grebing BR, Coughlin MJ. Evaluation of Morton's theory of second metatarsal hypertrophy. J Bone Joint Surg Am 2004;86-A(7):1375–86.
24. Wanivenhaus A, Pretterklieber M. First tarsometatarsal joint: anatomical biomechanical study. Foot Ankle Int 1989;9(4):153–7.
25. Hyer CF, Philbin TM, Berlet GC, et al. The incidence of the intermetatarsal facet of the first metatarsal and its relationship to metatarsus primus varus: a cadaveric study. J Foot Ankle Surg 2005;44(3):200–2.
26. Hyer CF, Philbin TM, Berlet GC, et al. The obliquity of the first metatarsal base. Foot Ankle Int 2004;25(10):728–32.
27. Bohne WH, Lee K-T, Peterson MG. Action of the peroneus longus tendon on the first metatarsal against metatarsus primus varus force. Foot Ankle Int 1997;18(8): 510–2.
28. Snijders C, Snijder J, Philippens M. Biomechanics of hallux valgus and spread foot. Foot Ankle 1986;7(1):26–39.
29. Grebing BR, Coughlin MJ. The effect of ankle position on the exam for first ray mobility. Foot Ankle Int 2004;25(7):467–75.
30. Mann RA, Katcherian DA. Relationship of metatarsophalangeal joint fusion on the intermetatarsal angle. Foot Ankle Int 1989;10(1):8–11.
31. Faber FW, Mulder PG, Verhaar JA. Role of first ray hypermobility in the outcome of the hohmann and the Lapidus procedure. A prospective, randomized trial involving one hundred and one feet. J Bone Joint Surg Am 2004;86-A(3):486–95.
32. Cronin JJ, Limbers JP, Kutty S, et al. Intermetatarsal angle after first metatarsophalangeal joint arthrodesis for hallux valgus. Foot Ankle Int 2006;27(2):104–9.
33. Grimes JS, Coughlin MJ. First metatarsophalangeal joint arthrodesis as a treatment for failed hallux valgus surgery. Foot Ankle Int 2006;27(11):887–93.

Hallux Valgus Deformity and Treatment

A Three-Dimensional Approach: Modified Technique for Lapidus Procedure

Robert D. Santrock, MD[a],*, Bret Smith, DO, MSc[b]

KEYWORDS

- Hallux valgus • Modified technique for Lapidus procedure • Classification system
- CORA • Triplane correction • Lapidus • Bunion

KEY POINTS

- It is without any doubt that the importance of triplane (transverse, sagittal, and frontal) correction of the hallux valgus (HAV) has become among the greatest improvements in bunion surgery.
- Triplane correction can be achieved reliably via first tarsometatarsal joint arthrodesis, the anatomic center of rotation of angulation (CORA) of the HAV deformity.
- Modified technique for Lapidus procedure (Treace Medical Concepts, Inc, Ponte Vedra Beach, FL, USA) is a surgical technique designed to incorporate triplane correction at the CORA of the HAV.
- A new classification system has been developed incorporating new three-dimensional computed tomography findings of HAV pathomechanics. It is hoped that this framework will provide further interest in research and discussion.
- The modified technique for Lapidus procedure can be used in a variety of HAV conditions and severities, and the early results suggest a powerful correction can be maintained.

INTRODUCTION

In a hallux valgus (HAV) or bunion deformity, the fundamental problem is deviation of the hallux at the metatarsophalangeal (MTP) joint and deviation of the first metatarsal at the tarsometatarsal (TMT) joint. Traditionally, anterior-posterior (AP) radiograph findings are prioritized, such as the intermetatarsal angle (IMA), the HAV angle (HVA), the tibial sesamoid position (TSP), and the joint surface angle known both as the distal metatarsal articular angle (DMAA) and the proximal articular set angle. It is vital to recognize

Disclosure Statement: All authors are consultants and design surgeons for Treace Medical Concepts, Inc.
[a] Department of Orthopaedics, West Virginia University, PO Box 9196, Morgantown, WV 26506-9196, USA; [b] Foot and Ankle Division, Moore Center for Orthopedics, Lexington, SC, USA
* Corresponding author.
E-mail address: rsantrock@hsc.wvu.edu

that, because the AP radiograph is a two-dimensional representation of the true three-dimensional anatomy, deviation in the other planes, such as frontal plane rotation of the first metatarsal, can substantially change all visible cues on an AP radiograph. Pronation of the first metatarsal changes the appearance of the DMAA, the TSP, the medial eminence, and the shape of the lateral metatarsal head. To identify and characterize the contribution of the frontal and sagittal plane deviations to the radiographic cues on the AP radiograph, different landmarks must be identified and the anatomy on axial and lateral radiographic views must be studied. This observation is important if one considers that the most prevalent methods recommended to correct the deformity (metatarsal osteotomy) are, in fact, altering a deviated but intrinsically straight metatarsal and are almost exclusively altering the transverse plane. Using only the traditional AP radiographic measurements to determine the surgical procedure is a potential primary factor driving poor outcomes and recurrence because the AP radiograph is not able to fully define the deformity. If most of the most popular osteotomy procedures are analyzed, it is clear that correction priority is in a single plane (transverse), with most procedures either angulating or sliding the first metatarsal in the transverse plane while failing to address either the frontal or sagittal planes to a meaningful degree.

In addition to recognizing the individual planar components, attention must be focused on the corrective procedure on the apex of the deformity or the anatomic center of rotation of angulation (CORA).[1] The apex of the metatarsal component of the deformity in a bunion has been described by many surgeons and researchers as being at the TMT joint, not in the metatarsal joint.[2–8] A published description of the frontal plane component of the first ray deformity dates back to the 1950s.[9] There are many current publications illustrating the effect that frontal plane rotation has on common paradigms of preoperative bunion evaluation and the selection of corrective procedure. In these studies, frontal plane rotation has consistently been observed to be in the direction of eversion (valgus or pronation are equivalent), having a significant and dramatic effect on the alignment of the first MTP joint, including the sesamoids.

The triplane TMT joint corrective arthrodesis, or modified technique for Lapidus procedure (Treace Medical Concepts, Ponte Vedra Beach, FL, USA), uses all 3 planes to both evaluate and correct the deformity. Interestingly, when this multiplanar technique is implemented, the traditional radiographic measurements become less useful. The idea that all bunions are different, and must be treated as such, is based on severity scales that are derived from AP radiographic measurements such as the IMA, the TSP, and the HVA. Using a triplane framework for evaluation and procedure selection, and focusing on the apex of the deformity, all bunions can be approached in a consistent manner. Specifically, the modified technique for Lapidus procedure can be performed regardless of the degree of deformity and always includes triplane correction. Big or small deformities become irrelevant when using this framework.

CLASSIFICATION

Classification systems for the HAV have historically been based on expert opinion with low levels of evidence and have focused mainly on two-dimensional radiographic observations. The angular measurements attempted to identify the degree of severity of the deformity and suggest possible corrective surgical measures. Classic radiographic findings such as the IMA, the HVA, and the sesamoid position have been identified by Laporta and colleagues.[10] These findings have all been substantiated in classic HAV textbooks.[11–15] Transverse plane considerations were also discussed by Meyr and colleagues.[16] In 2002, Condon and colleagues[17] described classic considerations in the HAV, referencing the IMA as normal (<9°), mild (9°–11°), moderate (11°–16°), and severe

(>16°). Based on the severity of the angle, various procedures are advocated that correlated to the anatomic location on the first metatarsal bone. A mild or low metatarsal 1-2 angle favors more distal osteotomies. More severe angles favor proximal procedures, and those with hypermobility include the Lapidus-type procedure.[11,18] Coughlin and Freund[19] analyzed the intraobserver and interobserver reliability of radiographic assessments of the HAV. Their study validated the reliability of the HVA and metatarsal 1-2 angles but questioned the DMAA. Garbuz and colleagues[20] stressed the importance of a valid classification system that has both intraobserver and interobserver reliability. Coughlin and Carlson[21] described angular osteotomies for the HAV associated with increased metatarsal 1-2 angle, the DMAA, and the proximal phalangeal articular angle.

In 2016, Deenik and colleagues[22] provided an excellent review of classification systems for the HAV. They found the only reliable assessment was the HVA. Despite the two-dimensional analysis and classifications to suggest surgical procedures, long-term clinical outcomes have not held up well over time, with recurrence rates from 25% to 65%.[23–26]

Since 2013, there has been an emergence of papers that have used weightbearing computed tomography studies that have provided an improved understanding of the pathomechanics of the HAV. These studies are a reminder to think in 3 dimensions and to consider the frontal plane component of HAV. The current frontal plane evaluation substantiates early observations by Morton[27] and Mizuno and colleagues,[9] and has been reported by numerous other investigators.[2,6,7,28–31]

With the advent of three-dimensional technology and other anatomic research, a new classification system known as the triplane hallux valgus classification (**Table 1**)

Table 1
Triplane hallux valgus classification

Class	Anatomic Findings	MTP Joint Status	Treatment Recommendation
1	Increased HVA and IMA No first metatarsal pronation evident on AP and sesamoid axial radiograph Sesamoids may be subluxed	No clinical or radiographic evidence of degenerative joint disease (DJD)	Transverse plane corrective procedure ± Distal soft tissue procedures
2A	Increased HVA and IMA First metatarsal pronation evident on AP and sesamoid axial radiograph No sesamoid subluxation on axial	No clinical or radiographic evidence of DJD	Triplane correction with first metatarsal supination or inversion
2B	Increased HVA and IMA First metatarsal pronation evident on AP and sesamoid axial radiograph With sesamoid subluxation on axial	No clinical or radiographic evidence of DJD	Triplane correction with first metatarsal supination or inversion Plus distal soft tissue procedures
3	Increased HVA and IMA >15° metatarsus adductus angle	No clinical or radiographic evidence of DJD	Metatarsal 2 and 3 transverse plane correction Followed by 1st metatarsal correction per class 1 & 2 recommendations
4	Increased HVA and IMA ± First metatarsal pronation	Clinical and/or radiographic evidence of DJD	First MTP joint arthrodesis

has been proposed. The uniqueness of this system is the lack of historical references to the angular severity of the deformity. It is based on surgical CORA and the angular correctional axis of the deformity. Even though the mechanical axis may be more proximal, the anatomic CORA is deemed more amenable for surgical repair that addresses transverse and sagittal plane hypermobility. It also takes into account whether pronation or eversion of the metatarsal segment (first ray) exists. Preoperative three-dimensional assessment is performed using at least AP, lateral, and axial radiographs.

No metatarsal rotation is found in class 1 that is amenable to shaft and base procedures for repair. This class is apparent in approximately 12.7% of HAV cases, as determined by Kim and colleagues.[29] In class 2, rotation is apparent and may exist with or without sesamoid subluxation (**Figs. 1** and **2**). Derotational procedures are performed with or without lateral sesamoid release. Rotational deformities occur in approximately 87.3% of the cases of HAV.[29] Class 3 identifies the unique attributes of metatarsal adductus that need to be addressed to achieve optimal results. The metatarsus adductus is a global forefoot deformity that usually requires basilar osteotomies of the second and third metatarsals, followed by correction of the first metatarsal to achieve optimal surgical repair. In this foot type, there is usually minimal eversion of the first metatarsal. Finally, class 4 incorporates arthrosis of the first metatarsal-phalangeal-sesamoid complex. Surgical procedures to address this condition are recommended and more commonly involve arthrodesis of the first metatarsal phalangeal joint. The goal of this classification is to provide a framework to assess the three-dimensional aspects of the HAV and to drive improvements in long-term outcomes.

PROCEDURE

The patient's operative extremity is marked and consent confirmed. For anesthesia, the authors' preference is a regional extremity nerve block performed by the anesthesia team. When the nerve block has been completed, the patient is taken to the operative suite and placed on a radiolucent operating room table. A tourniquet is

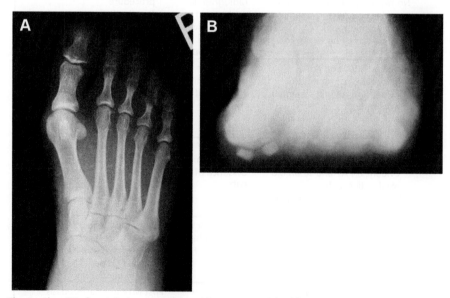

Fig. 1. Class 2A: frontal plane rotation without sesamoid subluxation. (*A*) Anterior-Posterior Weight-bearing Radiograph. (*B*) Axial Sesamoid Weight-bearing Radiograph.

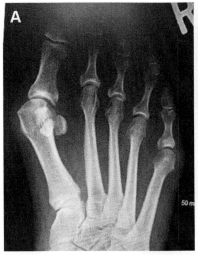
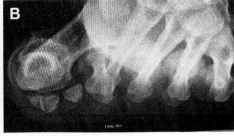

Fig. 2. Class 2B: frontal plane rotation with sesamoid subluxation. (*A*) Anterior-Posterior Weight-bearing Radiograph. (*B*) Axial Sesamoid Weight-bearing Radiograph.

applied to the operative limb and the limb is prepped and draped in the usual fashion for the operative procedure. The leg is exsanguinated and the tourniquet inflated to the appropriate pressure.

The initial incision is made over the dorsal aspect of the first TMT joint, just medial to the extensor hallucis longus tendon (**Fig. 3**). It is essential to keep the incision dorsal for this technique to allow the modified technique for Lapidus procedure system to work properly. The incision is developed until the dorsal aspect of the first TMT joint is exposed, then the entire dorsal and medial aspects of the joint are subperiosteally dissected.

Next, the joint is released to allow for rotation if a frontal plane deformity is noted preoperatively. The joint can be released plantarly using a combination of oscillating saw and osteotome (**Fig. 4**). A hemostat is used to open a small space at the proximal aspect of the first and second metatarsal interspace. A modified technique for Lapidus procedure fulcrum device is then placed into the interspace of the proximal first and second metatarsal (**Fig. 5**).

The mobility of the first MTP joint needs to be evaluated; if it is stiff or ankylosed, then a small webspace incision should be made and the tight lateral structures gradually released until the joint is mobilized. Importantly, opening the medial capsule of the first MTP joint should be avoided until the end of the case because destabilizing the medial structures will not allow the system to correct all 3 planes of the deformity properly. When the fulcrum has been placed, a modified technique for Lapidus procedure positioner device is ready to be applied. A small stab incision is made over the lateral portion of the second metatarsal, approximately 2.0 cm distal from the first TMT joint. The positioner is then applied distal to the fulcrum and the TMT joint (**Fig. 6**). The medial aspect of the positioner should be applied to the plantar medial ridge on the first metatarsal. The lateral portion of the positioner is placed over the lateral cortex of the second metatarsal.

Using the positioner, the HAV deformity can be corrected in all 3 planes. If the correction has been dialed into a satisfactory position, it can be confirmed on fluoroscopy. A Kirschner wire can be used to temporarily stabilize the corrected position with a pin placed through a cannulation in the positioner.

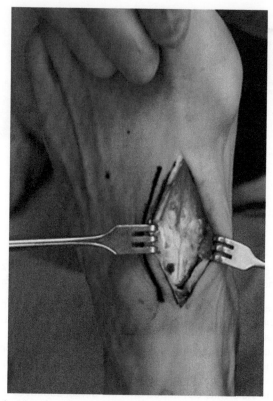

Fig. 3. The dorsal incision for the modified technique for Lapidus procedure technique.

The modified technique for Lapidus procedure joint seeker device is introduced dorsally in the first TMT joint, providing a placement guide for the cutting guide and assuring that the cuts are made correctly in the sagittal plane to prevent dorsiflexion of the first ray. The modified technique for Lapidus procedure cutting guide is placed over the joint seeker and temporarily fixed in place (**Fig. 7**). At this point, it is recommended to take an image with the C-arm to confirm alignment of the cutting guide. After the position has been confirmed, a final pin can be introduced to secure the

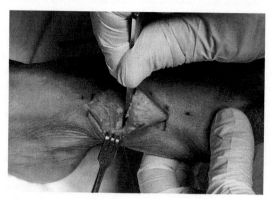

Fig. 4. Plantar capsular release using an osteotome.

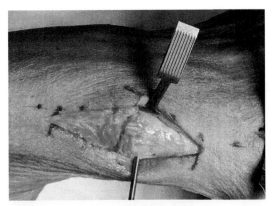

Fig. 5. Placement of the fulcrum between the bases of the first and second metatarsals.

cutting jig in position. The joint seeker is removed and the cuts on the base of the metatarsal and cuneiform can be completed.

The cut bone is removed using a combination of osteotome and rongeur. After all of the cut bone has been removed, the joint is prepared for arthrodesis. A drill bit is used to fenestrate the joint surfaces.

After the temporary holding pin in the positioner has been removed, the joint is axially compressed, held in the corrected position, and precompressed with the terminally threaded olive wire (**Fig. 8**). A second threaded olive wire can also be placed, based on surgeon preference. At this time, it is recommended to remove or release the positioner and check the correction with fluoroscopy.

If the position is satisfactory, final fixation can be applied. The current technique uses a Biplanar mini-plate construct, the Control 360 System (Treace Medical

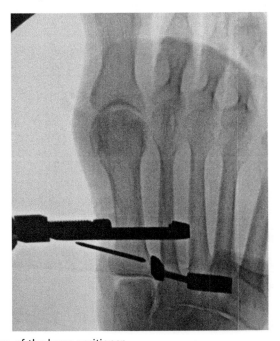

Fig. 6. Application of the bone positioner.

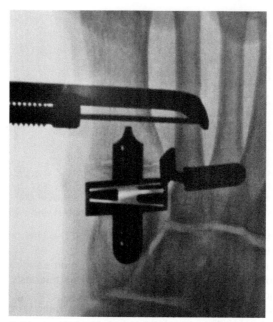

Fig. 7. Placement of the cut guide.

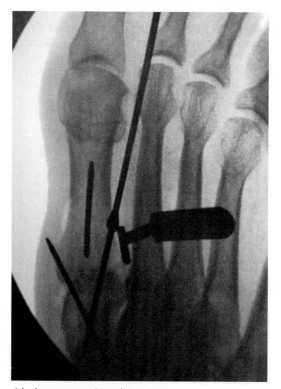

Fig. 8. Reduction with the compression olive wire.

Concepts, Ponte Vedra Beach, FL, USA), that offers multiplanar stability and allows for physiologic micromotion to promote healing as described by Perren.[32]

The initial plate is applied straight dorsal across the first TMT joint. After the plate is positioned, it is temporarily held in position with plate tacks. With the plate held in position, the other open holes are drilled in preparation for screw placement. The drill guides are removed and the locking screws are placed; the plate tacks can be removed and the final 2 locking screws are applied to the plate construct.

A second straight plate can be applied medially across the first TMT joint 90° to the dorsal plate, or a specially designed anatomic plantar-medial based plate, the Plantar Python Plate (Treace Medical Concepts, Ponte Vedra Beach, FL, USA), can be applied. As with the dorsal plate, the second plate is held with 2 plate tacks and then secured in sequence with the 4 locked screws (**Fig. 9**).

After the Biplanar plate construct has been applied, the surgeon does have the option of adding a screw from the first to the second metatarsal if there is suspicion of intercuneiform instability or if additional stabilization of the construct is desired.

After the first TMT joint has been stabilized, the surgeon can direct their attention to the first MTP joint. If needed, a medially based incision is used to access the joint. It is typically noted that there is significant capsular thickening that may require thinning. It is also not uncommon to find a dorsal ridge on the first metatarsal head that may also require removal.

After any additional procedures have been completed, the wounds are copiously irrigated and closed in the standard fashion. The patient is placed into a sterile dressing and either a stiffened postoperative shoe or low walking boot, based on surgeon preference.

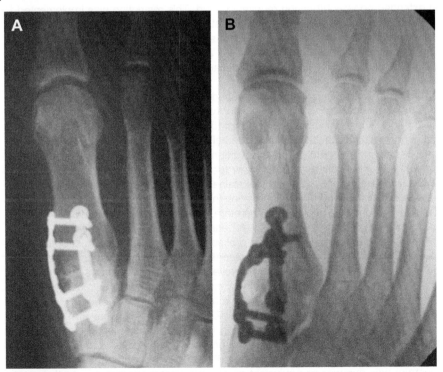

Fig. 9. Final construct (A) 90-90 Biplanar plating (B) Biplanar plating with plantar-medial Python plate.

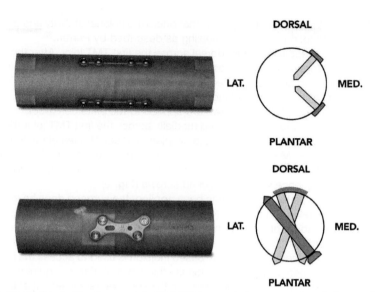

Fig. 10. Biomechanical testing models: 90-90 Biplanar plating versus dorsal plate with inter-fragmentary screw.

BIOMECHANICAL TESTING

One of the major hurdles that plagued the first TMT joint HAV corrections was the use of an extended nonweightbearing recovery period. This restriction was implemented to produce the most ideal situation for direct osteosynthesis (primary bone healing). Rigid fixation with zero to minimal micromotion is required for primary bone healing in a compression arthrodesis construct.[32] Zero micromotion is not normally compatible with weightbearing at the first TMT joint because there are significant deforming forces during gait.

The modified technique for Lapidus procedure system was designed to use secondary biological bone healing via relative stability fixation. This methodology has been well described by the AO (Arbeitsgemeinschaft für Osteosynthesefragen) Institute[32] and is the theory that drives the utilization of external fixation, intramedullary nails, and unicortical locking plate constructs. With this fixation, stability is achieved via multiplanar control, yet it is only relatively rigid to allow for controlled micromotion to stimulate the biological healing process. Perren[32] explained that this type of construct will produce bone healing via secondary bone formation through callous production as long as there is relative motion at the healing site. Therefore, a relative stability construct that has multiplanar stability may be more suitable for early to immediate weightbearing.

The modified technique for Lapidus procedure system has 2 construct options: unicortical Biplanar 90-90 construct or unicortical anatomic multiplanar construct with tension side (plantar) stabilization. However, the system is purposefully designed with relative rigidity to allow for some micromotion and, therefore, secondary bone formation. Both constructs have been biomechanically tested.

The original modified technique for Lapidus procedure Biplanar 90-90 construct was tested using cyclic cantilever loading to simulate immediate weightbearing. It was compared with a traditional Lapidus construct of a dorsal anatomic locking plate and interfragmentary compression screw (**Fig. 10**). In this comparison, the Biplanar construct was superior or equivalent in all force vector applications, both in static and fatigue testing (**Fig. 11**).[33]

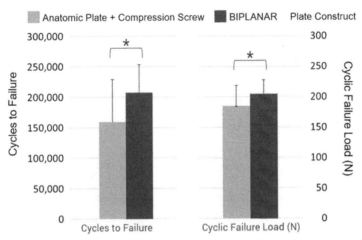

Fig. 11. Biomechanical results: 90-90 Biplanar plating versus dorsal plate and interfragmentary screw.

The modified technique for Lapidus procedure multiplanar construct was also tested in the same manner as the original Biplanar construct. The evolution of this construct is that 1 of the plates has an anatomic design purposely made to wrap to the tension (plantar) side of the first TMT joint arthrodesis site (**Fig. 12**), thus extending the stabilization at which the greatest forces are seen during gait. The results showed a superior performance of this anatomic tension side plate construct relative to the Biplanar 90-90 construct (**Fig. 13**).

EARLY CLINICAL AND RADIOGRAPHIC RESULTS

The traditional drawback of the Lapidus procedure is the need for extended immobilization; recent studies have challenged this standard with weightbearing beginning at 2 to 3 weeks.[34,35] (**) However, with the biomechanical evidence previously presented, the goal was to push the weightbearing to immediately postoperative.

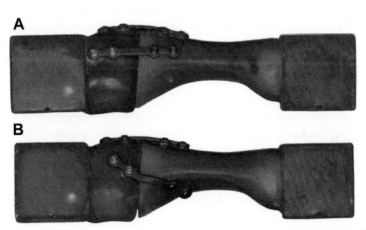

Fig. 12. Biomechanical testing models: 90-90 Biplanar plating versus Biplanar plating with plantar-medial python plate.

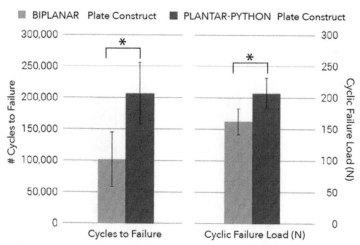

Fig. 13. Biomechanical results: 90-90 Biplanar plating versus Biplanar plating with plantar-medial python plate.

A multicenter study of subjects who underwent modified technique for Lapidus procedure and were treated with immediate weightbearing was presented to the American Orthopedic Foot and Ankle Society.[36] The objective of the study was to perform an early evaluation of this novel procedure that allowed for triplane correction and immediate weightbearing after Lapidus arthrodesis. The study had 4 centers and the subjects were collected consecutively, excluding revision cases, multiple simultaneous arthrodesis (ie, transverse midfoot fusions), and severe degenerative joint disease at the first MTP joint. There was a minimum 3-month follow-up to review for radiographic evidence of recurrence, hardware failure, or nonunion. The study also collected complications such as delayed wound healing and hardware removal. Forty-nine symptomatic HAV subjects (average age 41.9 ± 17.9 years; follow-up 4.3 ± 1.0 months) were collected. Both fixation construct options described in the previous section were used in this study. The first plating construct (28 of 49 subjects) placed 1 straight plate on the dorsal surface and another straight plate on the medial surface, 90° to each other. The second multiplanar construct (21 of 49 subjects) placed a straight plate on the dorsal surface and the anatomic tension-side plate

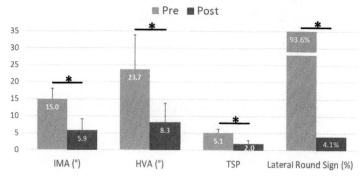

Fig. 14. Preoperative and postoperative radiographic results of immediate weightbearing after modified technique for Lapidus procedure.

Table 2
Complications following immediate weightbearing

Delayed wound healing or swelling	2 (4%)
Broken screw in fixation construct	1 (2%)
Hardware removal for soft-tissue irritation	1 (2%)
Undercorrection (IMA >10° or HVA >20°)	2 (4%)
Nonunion	0 (0%)

from the medial surface of the cuneiform to the plantar surface of the first metatarsal. For the postoperative regimen, all subjects were placed into a toe-spica dressing with a rigid-bottom shoe or boot, and allowed immediate weightbearing as tolerated. Preoperative and final postoperative radiographs were measured to assess the 1-2 IMA, the HVA, the lateral shape of the metatarsal head (lateral round sign), and the TSP, which was measured using the Hardy and Clapham[37] 1 to 7 scale. Additionally, the final postoperative radiographs were reviewed for assessment of radiographic fusion. Paired t-tests were conducted to determine the change in the anatomic radiographic measures. The radiographic results demonstrated a significant improvement in the IMA, the HVA, and the TSP (**Fig. 14**). Elimination of the metatarsal round sign, indicating correction of frontal-plane metatarsal rotation, was observed in 47 of the 49 feet (95.9%). Under the immediate protected weightbearing protocol, 0 of the 49 feet (0%) demonstrated evidence of nonunion at final follow-up. Regarding complications, there were 2 cases (4.1%) of undercorrection and 1 case (2.0%) of hardware removal for soft tissue irritation (**Table 2**). The results of the study support the hypothesis that immediate weightbearing is possible following first TMT joint fusion with 2 low-profile, unicortical locking plates at 90° orientation without an interfragmentary screw. These results demonstrated maintenance of the triplane correction without increased risk of nonunion.

As of July 2017, more than 1500 modified technique for Lapidus procedure HAV corrections had been performed.

ACKNOWLEDGMENTS

Daniel J. Hatch, DPM, FACFAS, and Paul Dayton, DPM, MS, FACFAS, contributed to this article.

REFERENCES

1. Paley D. Radiographic assessment of lower limb deformities. In: Principles of deformity correction. Heidelberg (Germany): Springer; 2002. p. 31–60.
2. Mortier J-P, Bernard J-L, Maestro M. Axial rotation of the first metatarsal head in a normal population and hallux valgus patients. Orthop Traumatol Surg Res 2012; 98:677–83.
3. Tanaka Y, Takakura Y, Sugimoto K, et al. Precise anatomic configuration changes in the first ray of the hallux valgus foot. Foot Ankle Int 2000;21:651–6.
4. King DM, Toolan BC. Associated deformities and hypermobility in hallux valgus: an investigation with weightbearing radiographs. Foot Ankle Int 2004;25:251–5.
5. Vyas S, Conduah A, Vyas N, et al. The role of the first metarsocuneiform joint in juvenile hallux valgus. J Pediatr Orthop B 2010;19:399–402.
6. Dayton P, Feilmeier M, Kauwe M, et al. Relationship of frontal plane rotation of first metatarsal to proximal articular set angle and hallux alignment in patients

undergoing tarsometatarsal arthrodesis for hallux abducto valgus: a case series and critical review of the literature. J Foot Ankle Surg 2013;52:348–54.

7. Okuda R, Yasuda T, Jotoku T, et al. Proximal abduction-supination osteotomy of the first metatarsal for adolescent hallux valgus: a preliminary report. J Orthop Sci 2013;18:419–25.

8. DiDomenico LA, Fahim R, Rollandini J, et al. Correction of frontal plane rotation of sesamoid apparatus during the Lapidus procedure: a novel approach. J Foot Ankle Surg 2014;53:248–51.

9. Mizuno S, Sima Y, Yamazaki K. Detorsion osteotomy of the first metatarsal bone in hallux valgus. J Jpn Orthop Assoc 1956;30:813–9.

10. Laporta G, Melillo T, Olinsky D. X-ray evaluation of hallux abducto valgus deformity. J Am Podiatry Assoc 1974;64:544–66.

11. Coughlin MJ, Mann RA. Hallux valgus and complications of the hallux. In: Mann RA, editor. Surgery of the foot and ankle. St Louis (MO): CV Mosby; 1986. p. 65–131.

12. Inman VT. DuVries' surgery of the foot. St Louis (MO): Mosby; 1973.

13. Kelikian H. Hallux valgus, allied deformities of the forefoot and metatarsalgia. Philadelphia: Saunders; 1965.

14. Palladino SJ. Preoperative evaluation of the bunion patient. In: Gerbert J, editor. Textbook of bunion surgery. Third edition. Philadelphia: W.B. Saunders; 2001. p. 3–71.

15. Ruch J, Banks A. First ray hallux abducto valgus and related deformities. In: Dalton McGlammry E, editor. Comprehensive textbook of foot surgery. Baltimore (MD): Williams and Wilkins; 1987. p. 144–50.

16. Meyr AJ, Myers A, Pontious J. Descriptive quantitative analysis of hallux abductovalgus transverse plane radiographic parameters. J Foot Ankle Surg 2014;53: 397–404.

17. Condon F, Kaliszer M, Conhyea D, et al. The first intermetatarsal angle in hallux valgus: an analysis of measurement reliability and the error involved. Foot Ankle Int 2002;23:717–21.

18. Robinson AHN, Limbers JP. Modern concepts in the treatment of hallux valgus. J Bone Joint Surg Br 2005;87:1038–45.

19. Coughlin MJ, Freund E. The reliability of angular measurements in hallux valgus deformities. Foot Ankle Int 2001;22:369–79.

20. Garbuz DS, Masri BA, Esdaile J, et al. Classification systems in orthopaedics. J Am Acad Orthop Surg 2002;10:290.

21. Coughlin MJ, Carlson RE. Treatment of hallux valgus with an increased distal metatarsal articular angle: evaluation of double and triple first ray osteotomies. Foot Ankle Int 1999;20:762–70.

22. Deenik A, Verburg A, Louwerens JW, et al. Evidence of treatment algorithms for hallux valgus. JSM Foot and Ankle 2016;1(1):1–6.

23. Agrawal Y, Desai A, Mehta J. Lateral sesamoid position in hallux valgus: correlation with the conventional radiological assessment. Foot Ankle Surg 2011;17: 308–11.

24. Bock P, Kluger R, Kristen K-H, et al. The scarf osteotomy with minimally invasive lateral release for treatment of hallux valgus deformity. J Bone Joint Surg Am 2015;97:1238–45.

25. Iyer S, Demetracopoulos CA, Sofka CM, et al. High rate of recurrence following proximal medial opening wedge osteotomy for correction of moderate hallux valgus. Foot Ankle Int 2015;36:756–63.

26. Raikin SM, Miller AG, Daniel J. Recurrence of hallux valgus: a review. Foot Ankle Clin 2014;19:259–74.
27. Morton DJ. Metatarsus atavicus. J Bone Joint Surg 1927;9:531–4.
28. Bradley C, Miller M, Conti S. Pronation of the first metatarsal in hallux valgus. Presented at the Orthopedic Research Society, San Diego, March 14-18, 2017.
29. Kim Y, Kim JS, Young KW, et al. A new measure of tibial sesamoid position in hallux valgus in relation to the coronal rotation of the first metatarsal in CT scans. Foot Ankle Int 2015;36:944–52.
30. Scranton PE Jr, Rutkowski R. Anatomic variations in the first ray: part I. Anatomic aspects related to bunion surgery. Clin Orthop Relat Res 1980;151:244–55.
31. Talbot KD, Saltzman CL. Assessing sesamoid subluxation: how good is the AP radiograph? Foot Ankle Int 1998;19:547–54.
32. Perren SM. Evolution of the internal fixation of long bone fractures. The scientific basis of biological internal fixation: choosing a new balance between stability and biology. J Bone Joint Surg Br 2002;84B:1093–110.
33. Dayton P, Ferguson J, Hatch DJ, et al. Comparison of the mechanical characteristics of a universal small biplane plating technique without compression screw and single anatomic plate with compression screw. J Foot Ankle Surg 2016;55:567–71.
34. Sorensen MD, Hyer CF, Berlet GC. Results of lapidus arthrodesis and locked plating with early weight bearing. Foot Ankle Spec 2009;2:227–33.
35. Prissel MA, Hyer CF, Grambart ST, et al. A multicenter, retrospective study of early weightbearing for modified lapidus arthrodesis. J Foot Ankle Surg 2016;55:226–9.
36. Smith WB, Santrock RD, Hatch D, et al. Immediate weight bearing after biplanar plantar fixation of lapidus: a multi-centered study. AOFAS Annual Meeting, Seattle, WA, March 14-18, 2017.
37. Hardy RH, Clapham JC. Observations on hallux valgus; based on a controlled series. J Bone Joint Surg Br 1951;33:376–91.

Hallux Valgus/Medial Column Instability and Their Relationship with Posterior Tibial Tendon Dysfunction

Steven Blackwood, MD[a],*, Leland Gossett, MD[b]

KEYWORDS

- Bunions • Flat foot deformity • Adult acquired flatfoot deformity
- Posterior tibial tendon dysfunction • Hallux valgus • Medial column instability

KEY POINTS

- Historically, bunions have focused on the coronal plane; however, there is tension and compression failure in the sagittal plane of the midfoot during arch collapse.
- Correction of all 3 planes of deformity: coronal, sagittal, and rotational, can be achieved in several ways.
- Taking a big picture of global foot mechanics by recognizing the common types of conditions associated with arch collapse, including hallux valgus deformities, can serve as a useful roadmap for navigating more complicated deformities where hallux valgus exists.

INTRODUCTION

Before 1980,[1] acquired flatfoot deformity was thought to be quite rare, but considerable attention has been directed to recognizing and treating the various stages of pathology of a condition now considered common. The posterior tibial tendon itself has been the focus of most research and its failure is traditionally regarded as a causal factor of the adult acquired flatfoot deformity. A greater understanding of the individual components that together contribute to the clinical appearance of the flatfoot and surgery is now individualized based on correcting each component of the deformity. In 1989, Johnson and Strom[2] solidified the general understanding of dysfunction of the posterior tibial tendon (PTT), and this condition remains synonymous with the various stages of adult acquired flatfoot deformity (AAFD). As the understanding of

Disclosure: The authors have nothing to disclose.
[a] Orthopaedic Associates of Michigan, 1111 Leffingwell Avenue NE, Grand Rapids, MI 49525, USA; [b] Spectrum Health - Michigan State University, 221 Michigan Street NE, Suite 402, Grand Rapids, MI 49503, USA
* Corresponding author.
E-mail address: steven.blackwood@gmail.com

PTT dysfunction (PTTD) and AAFD has continued to expand, it has been stated that adult acquired flatfoot is too complex to be classified as a simply different stage of PTTD.[3] However, with a greater awareness of attention to the atavistic human tendency toward equinus-driven collapse, the understanding of the pathomechanics of the acquired flexible flatfoot deformity has matured. The term equinus never appears in the Johnson and Strom[4] article; however, it is accepted that a heel cord contracture is an integral consideration of the overall deformity and should be addressed in most if not all reconstructions.[5,6]

BIOMECHANICS OF POSTERIOR TIBIAL TENDON AND ARCH SUPPORT

Stabilization of the longitudinal arch by the PTT continues to be debated, and there is support for both static and dynamic stabilization. Static support theorists fall into 2 camps: those believing the foot acts as a truss, and those believing the foot acts as a beam. The truss theory is supported by Lapidus.[4] A truss works by creating 2 struts that meet at an apex, supported at the base by a tie rod, thus forming a triangle. As the apex is loaded, compressive forces are applied to the struts, and tensile forces are applied to the tie rod. As long as the tie rod remains intact, the struts do not collapse, and the truss holds firm. Relating this model to the anatomy of the foot, the tie rod becomes the plantar aponeurosis and plantar supporting ligaments. Hicks[7,8] believes that this model becomes critical at toe-off, when the windlass mechanism has maximal effect.

HALLUX VALGUS AS A MULTIPLANAR DEFORMITY

Although hallux valgus is most simply described and understood as a two-dimensional transverse plane deformity of the first metatarsal, it is more accurately a triplanar deformity consisting deviation in the transverse, sagittal, and frontal planes. In our classification, we view hallux valgus as a manifestation of tension failure in progressive arch collapse. Although first ray instability can present as isolated sagittal plane or dorsal instability, it more commonly occurs as multiplanar dorsomedial instability leading to hallux valgus. In a study of 600 feet, Singh and colleagues[9,10] reported increased dorsal (7.2 vs 9.8 mm) and 45° dorsomedial (8.3 vs 11.0 mm) instability in patients with hallux valgus.[11] This is in keeping with biomechanical and anatomic studies. The first metatarsal–cuneiform joint axis is approximately 45 to 60° angled dorsomedially from the horizontal. This axis of motion is likely to accommodate foot pronation through toe-off, but may help explain this common pattern of instability and its implication in the development of hallux valgus. In our series of outcomes on 412 Lapidus procedures performed for a spectrum of forefoot pathologies, 62% had concomitant modified McBride procedures for hallux valgus whereas 90% of patients had documented first ray hypermobility on examination.[12] This implies that dorsomedial instability is the more common instability pattern seen at the first ray.[12] Finally, the third plane of metatarsal deformity in hallux valgus involves metatarsal pronation. This rotational deformity seems to be clearly correlated with progression of first ray instability and arch collapse. In 1 radiographic study of 50 weight-bearing feet, there was a linear negative correlation between first metatarsal pronation and height of the medial longitudinal arch.[13] In fact, this correlation was stronger than that observed between pronation and increased intermetatarsal angle.[13] Due to established descriptions of hallux valgus predominantly on transverse plane measurements, it is likely that this deformity is underappreciated. In one series of feet treated with Lapidus and modified McBride procedures, a significant reduction in proximal articular set angle was seen despite no distal bony realignment procedures performed.[14] In the same series, Dayton and colleagues[14] reported significant reduction of medial eminence size without bony resection. The investigators concluded that both of these metrics viewed as transverse plane deformities of the distal metatarsal are more accurately radiographic artifacts of morphologically normal metatarsals viewed obliquely due to rotational deformity.[14] It is our view that a first tarsometatarsal (TMT) arthrodesis is superior to commonly used corrective metatarsal osteotomies in its ability to address all 3 of these deformities.

ADDITIONAL DEFORMING FORCES IN HALLUX VALGUS

An expansion of the tibialis posterior tendon into the short flexor and oblique adductor of the big toe was found as a constant anatomic variation in the feet of cadavers with hallux valgus deformities. This expansion was not found in dissected normal feet. This expansion may be considered as a contributive factor, among other factors, in the etiology of hallux valgus deformities.[15] This anomalous structure has continued to be discussed by Gunal and colleagues,[16] in 1994, and shows the dynamic role of anomalous expansions of the tibialis posterior tendon into the oblique part of adductor hallucis muscle in patients with hallux valgus. We suggest this expansion be excised in addition to other operative procedures selected for the surgical treatment of patients with hallux valgus.[16]

In addition to this variation of the PTT, there is additional anatomic explanation linking the pathogenesis of hallux valgus to the development of arch collapse. In a cadaveric study, Wong[17] found that the abductor hallucis has a consistent fascial sling in the hindfoot and insertion through the tibial sesamoid. Simulated contraction of this muscle leads to flexion and supination of the first metatarsal, elevating the arch and resisting the deformity of hallux valgus. In addition to the role of extrinsics, such as the gastrocnemius, in driving equinus and the PTT in resisting hindfoot deformity, the abductor hallucis may contribute as an intrinsic muscle implicated in the development of hallux valgus.[17]

LOOK AT THE WHOLE PICTURE

The most widely accepted paradigm for arch collapse results from the Johnson and Strom 1989 publication discussed previously. The Johnson classification is categorized into 4 classes: type 1: no deformity, type 2: flexible deformity, type 3: fixed deformity, type 4: ankle deformity. Although this is an oversimplification of the Johnson classification, the classification is still relying on the concept that it is the results of posterior tibialis tendon insufficiency.

In 1999, Anderson and Hansen[11] reviewed the pathomechanics of Type 2 PTTD and included what they termed an "alternative scenario." In this scenario, equinus deformity contributes to the driving force involved in failure of the medial column. An isolated contracture of the gastrocnemius or a combined gastrocsoleus complex contracture causes increased stress on the medial longitudinal arch. Strain is transmitted across the entire medial column: talonavicular, naviculocuneiform, and TMT articulations. Ligamentous supports stretch, allowing forefoot supination. This deformity progresses to involve the hindfoot once the spring ligament becomes attenuated. The end result of the unstable medial column is hindfoot valgus. This cascade of events causes progressive PTTD, resulting from a new line of pull and greater excursion requirements on the posterior tibialis.

The new paradigm is that arch collapse can occur without PTT pathology. The arch collapses in a sequential and predictable manner with multiple clinical entities involved. Given these findings, a new classification is needed for a more complete understanding and evaluation of arch collapse and associated findings.

Our classification (**Table 1**) is one of progressive arch collapse, driven by gravity and equinus, and presents a new approach to evaluating arch collapse. Biomechanically, the foot acts as a tripod and requires a stable medial column. The legs of this tripod are made up of the first ray, fifth ray, and heel. As body weight comes down on the talus, the forces are distributed across the foot. The natural reaction force is for the medial arch to collapse, indicated by an elevation of the first ray axis relative to the talar declination seen in the lateral plane. This collapse leads to failure in compression dorsally and in tension on the plantar aspect. Normally, collapse is prevented by the surrounding ligaments and plantar fascia. When the medial longitudinal arch collapses, the first ray begins to elevate, leading to biomechanical changes in the way the foot accepts weight. Once the spring ligament attenuates, the talonavicular joint subluxes, the talar head becomes uncovered, and the heel begins to tip into valgus (**Fig. 1**).

Figs. 2 and **3** show an example of a normal weight-bearing anteroposterior and lateral radiograph of the foot. Note the linear relationship between the talus and the first metatarsal on both anteroposterior and lateral radiographs. The medial longitudinal arch is intact. The first metatarsal is centered over the sesamoid bones. There is a smooth transitional parabola along the metatarsal heads.

Table 1
The Grand Rapids Arch Collapse Classification (GRACC)

Classification	Affected Part of the Foot	Presenting Pathology	Biomechanics
Type 1	Gastrocnemius (precollapse, no foot deformity)	• Gastrocnemius equinus • Plantar fasciitis • Metatarsalgia • Achilles tendon pain	• Weakened support of the arches • Tensile failure of posterior and plantar soft tissues
Type 2	Forefoot	• Hypermobile first ray • Hallux valgus • Lesser toe deformity • Metatarsalgia • Metatarsal stress fracture	• Medial column incompetence with weight-bearing transfer to lesser rays
Type 3	Midfoot	• Midfoot arthritis: 　○ Second and third tarsometatarsal arthritis 　○ Medial navicular arthritis	• Transverse arch collapse
Type 4	Hindfoot	• Hindfoot valgus • Peritalar subluxation • Posterior tibial tendon pathology • Lateral hindfoot/subtalar arthritis • Sinus tarsi impingement	• Medial arch collapse with spring ligament attenuation and hindfoot valgus
Type 5	Ankle	• Valgus ankle arthritis	• Deltoid ligament attenuation

From Anderson JG, Bohay DR, Eller EB, et al. Gastrocnemius Recession. Foot Ankle Clin N Am 2014; 19:4;767–86; with permission.

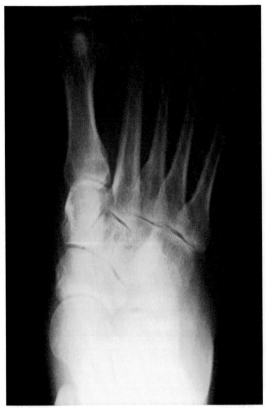

Fig. 1. Weight-bearing anteroposterior radiograph view of flatfoot collapse (type IV GRACC). Note the talar head uncovering.

As the first ray becomes more mobile, the deviation of the first metatarsal has increased in the coronal plane. The sesamoids are more uncovered. The tensile side of the first TMT joint has started to show some gapping, evidence now of hypermobility of the first TMT joint in both coronal and sagittal planes (**Figs. 4** and **5**).

Compare this to a flatfoot deformity, seen in **Figs. 6–8**. Note the medial column collapse that has occurred at the first TMT joint, the naviculocuneiform (NC) and the talonavicular joint. The first ray has elevated, evidence of a hypermobile first ray and the hindfoot has tilted into valgus. The talar head becomes uncovered as the spring ligament becomes attenuated. In other words, the tripod has tipped over.

The Grand Rapids Arch Collapse Classification (GRACC) (see **Table 1**) was designed to highlight the progressive collapse of the arch, noted with tensile failure of the plantar soft tissues and compression failure of the dorsal midfoot joints. Please see (**Figs. 6** and **8**) for a clinical demonstration of the arch collapse.

A GRACC type I involves a precollapse condition with a gastrocnemius contracture leading to midfoot and forefoot overload. The patient presents with pain, typically on the plantar or posterior aspect, involving the soft tissues loaded in tension. Associated findings in this type as a result of the gastroc contracture include Achilles tendinopathy, plantar fasciitis, metatarsalgia, and arch pain without radiographic abnormality. With persistent gastrocnemius contracture, the arch begins to collapse with forefoot deformity, denoting a Grand Rapids type II.

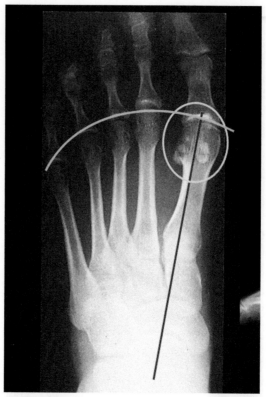

Fig. 2. Weight-bearing anteroposterior radiograph view of a normal foot. Note the normal cascade of metatarsal heads, the alignment of the talar head with the first metatarsal and sesamoids are seated under the first metatarsal head.

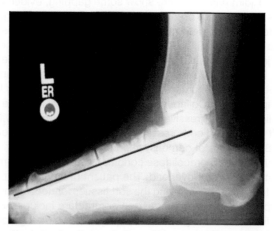

Fig. 3. Weight-bearing lateral radiograph view of a normal foot. The blue line shows the normal alignment of the medial column with the talus in line with the first metatarsal.

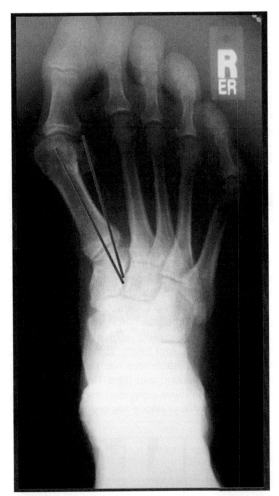

Fig. 4. Weight-bearing anteroposterior radiograph view of a hypermobile first ray. The medial blue line follows the anatomic axis of the first metatarsal. The lateral blue line shows where a normal first metatarsal would be located.

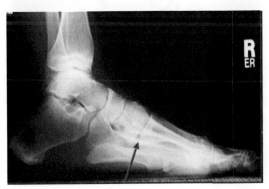

Fig. 5. Weight-bearing lateral radiograph view showing plantar gapping of the first tarso-metatarsal jointm representing an unstable joint.

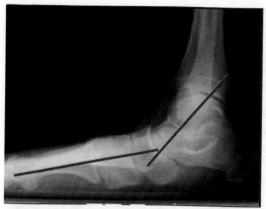

Fig. 6. Non–weight-bearing lateral radiograph views of flatfoot deformity. The blue lines show arch collapse with an increase Meary's angle as the first ray elevates.

This continued overload creates hypermobility in the first TMT joint and first ray elevation. This hypermobility can bring about further forefoot deformities, including hallux valgus. Furthermore, the unstable first TMT joint leads to an overload of the lesser metatarsals, causing metatarsalgia, intractable plantar keratoses, metatarso-phalangeal joint synovitis, and hammer toe deformities.

Less commonly, dorsiflexion/compression stress at the lesser TMT joints leads to midfoot arthritis rather than the forefoot failing at the metatarsophalangeal joints. A Grand Rapids type III deformity characterizes such a midfoot deformity. The typical pattern of arthritis involves the second and third TMT joints and progresses to the medial naviculocuneiform joint in more advanced midfoot deformity. Type III defor-mities are often precipitated by a previous history of bunion pain, metatarsalgia,

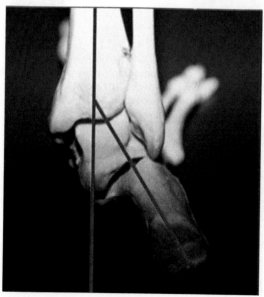

Fig. 7. Clinical demonstration of arch collapse, change plantar to posterior view. As the tripod collapses medially, the hindfoot goes into valgus.

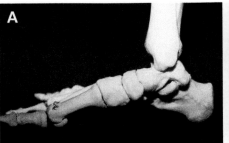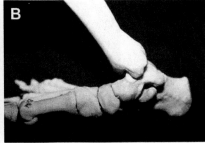

Fig. 8. (*A*) Normal arch with weight bearing. (*B*) Clinical example of how the arch of the foot fails. Note compression failure dorsally and tension failure plantarly. (*Courtesy of* Orthopaedic Associates of Michigan, Grand Rapids, MI.)

hammertoes, arch pain, plantar fasciitis, or Achilles tendon pathology, but have now progressed to dorsal compressive failure of the midfoot joints, with associated arthritis and dorsal osteophytes and joint space loss.

As the arch continues to collapse, further elevation of the first ray can produce spring ligament attenuation leading to lateral or dorsolateral peritalar subluxation and subsequent hindfoot valgus deformity. This hindfoot valgus pathology is the defining characteristic of the Grand Rapids type IV deformity. It is in the type IV deformity that PTTD is typically found, due to spring ligament attenuation and resulting dorsal and lateral subluxation of the navicular around the talar head with talar head uncoverage (**Fig. 9**). It is in this clinical environment where the workload on the posterior tibialis is increased (work equals force × distance) as a result of the increased excursion on the PTT when the navicular subluxes laterally.

Finally, with continued valgus malalignment of the hindfoot, in concert with the attenuation of the deltoid ligament, valgus deformity and degenerative joint changes of the tibiotalar joint are the primary traits of a GRACC type V deformity, the final type of arch collapse.

For the purposes of this article, we focus on the GRACC II, III, and IV types of arch collapse that are associated with hallux valgus: tight gastrocnemius with medial column breakdown, and associated isolated forefoot, midfoot, and hindfoot problems.

IDEAL PROCEDURE FOR HALLUX VALGUS

The ideal procedure for hallux valgus corrects the deformity where it originates. The bony structures of the first ray do not become crooked, but rather the deformity originates at the first TMT joint. The first TMT joint does not have any inherent stability because it is a uniplanar joint and there is no 1 to 2 intermetatarsal ligament. The typical hallux valgus deformity is associated with a metatarsus primus varus, which leads to uncovering of the sesamoids. Correction of multiplanar deformity is best done by correcting coronal, sagittal, and rotational planes. While correcting the hallux valgus angle, the surgeon is also making certain that the first ray is down even with the second and third metatarsal heads. Shortening of the first ray can have deleterious effects postoperatively, as this can lead to transfer lesions. The goal should be to ensure that all 6 points of contact in the forefoot weight-bearing bones (2 sesamoids and each of the 4 lesser metatarsal heads) strike the ground at the same time and distribute force equally. One can minimize shortening by exposing only subchondral bone and doing minimal bone resection to correct varus at the TMT joint. If excessive shortening exists, or a preexisting transfer lesion exists, then one should consider shortening the

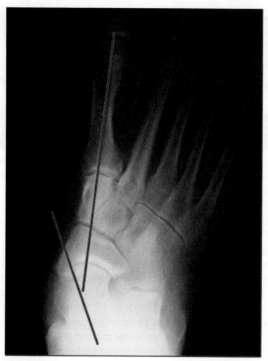

Fig. 9. Non–weight-bearing anteroposterior radiograph view of flatfoot deformity. This radiograph represents a GRACC type IV with talar head uncovering and loss of alignment between the talar head and first metatarsal. The talar head uncovering would indicate a spring ligament disruption.

second metatarsal and possibly further adjacent metatarsals to keep the relative lengthens satisfactory.

OUTCOMES OF TARSOMETATARSAL FUSION FOR HALLUX VALGUS

The Lapidus procedure has long been a favored technique for severe deformity correction or revision surgery for failed or recurrent deformity. This has been confirmed by multiple studies. In a large symptomatic review of multiple techniques, intermetatarsal angle correction 8.5 to 14.4° was noted depending on fixation technique with an overall fusion rate of 4%.[18] It is our view that when done correctly, the modified Lapidus procedure is an ideal technique for hallux valgus correction in most circumstances.

A major criticism of using first TMT arthrodesis as a primary option for hallux valgus correction is the historically high rate of nonunion. Nonunion rates have ranged from 0% to 12%, with revision rates for symptomatic nonunions ranging from 0% to 7.5%[19,20]; however, operative techniques in these reports were varied, and many were outdated. In our review of the literature from the past 3 decades, we found a wide range of reported operative techniques. First, joint preparation was largely carried out with saw resection. Second, joint fenestration was not uniformly performed. Third, joint fixation was highly variable, with many investigators using constructs relying on K-wire or Steinmann pin fixation.[19] There are several more recent reports from a variety of institutions confirming that expected rates of fusion with modern operative techniques far exceed those historically reported. Mani and colleagues[21] reported in 2015 a 2.7% nonunion rate with crossed screw fixation and interpositional autograft in 182 feet. Barp and colleagues[22] published a comparative study of fusion rates with multiple fixation techniques and found a 6.7% overall fusion rate with 4% rate of revision fusion. They reported a trend toward highest risk of nonunion and lowest need for hardware removal with crossed screw fixation.[14] Finally, in a 2015 meta-analysis, Donnenwerth and colleagues[23] reported on an aggregate nonunion rate of 5% with a symptomatic rate of 56%.

Compared with historical methods, modern techniques rely more frequently on indwelling hardware, which poses the risk of symptomatic hardware. Peterson and colleagues[19] reported on a series of 165 consecutive patients and found a 15% rate of symptomatic hardware at 9 months postoperatively after Lapidus fusion with dorsomedial locking plate. Although this is a concern, it is our experience that crossed screw fixation without supplementary plate fixation does not routinely require reoperation for symptomatic hardware.

The second major criticism with first TMT arthrodesis is the long period of postoperative non–weight bearing historically required to achieve union. Again, although a period of non–weight bearing is still standard practice, this is likely based on the historical use of fixation constructs that were inadequate to allow for early mobilization and weight bearing. Several recent reports have challenged the necessity for a prolonged period of postoperative non-weight bearing while maintaining excellent rates of union. In a series by King and colleagues,[24] 136 patients underwent a modified Lapidus procedure with crossed screw fixation, with protected weight bearing initiated at an average of 12 days postoperative, with full weight bearing at an average of 34 days postoperative. They reported a nonunion rate of 2.2%, with a symptomatic nonunion rate of 1.5% and no increased risk of malunion or other complications. In another recent series, first TMT fusion was performed using a plantar compression plate construct. Seventeen patients were allowed immediate full weight bearing in a postoperative shoe and compared with 17 patients who were kept non–weight bearing for 6 weeks postoperatively. They reported no increase in the rate of complications and earlier return to work in the group allowed immediate weight bearing.[25] Furthermore, recent reports suggest boot or cast immobilization may not be necessary either. Kazzaz and Singh[26] reported on a consecutive series of 27 feet managed in a postoperative wedge shoe and found no nonunions.

Although there is ample evidence confirming the effectiveness of first metatarsal arthrodesis for deformity correction and pain reduction, there exists the theoretic concern that midfoot fusion could alter foot mechanics and limit high-level activity. However, MacMahon and colleagues[27] reported on a cohort of 58 young physically active patients on their return to activity after undergoing first TMT fusion. They found 40% of patients returned to activity at a higher level than preoperatively, whereas 41% were equivalent and 19% had some level impairment to participation. Overall, they conclude that the modified Lapidus procedure is a viable option for hallux valgus correction in young active patients wishing to return to sport.

TARSOMETATARSAL FUSIONS

Our preferred technique for treatment of medial column instability in the setting of a type II GRACC is a TMT fusion. This is typically accomplished with two 3.5-mm cortical lag screws and supplemented with local bone graft as "spot weld" to help promote union. Our current technique also routinely includes arthrodesis between the first and second metatarsals, and screw fixation between the medial and middle cuneiforms with or without formal joint preparation. In our experience, bony fusion between the first and second ray is reliably achieved using this method, ensuring against recurrence of metatarsus primus adductus and hallux valgus deformities.

Previous criticisms of the modified Lapidus procedure have been prolonged convalescence, unacceptable nonunion rates, shortening and dorsal drift of the first ray, and transfer metatarsalgia. Reported outcomes have been consistently good to excellent in 70% to 92% of patients.[28-31] In our 2005 publication, when including all patients undergoing a first TMT joint arthrodesis as part of a modified Lapidus or as part of a flatfoot reconstruction, we were able to critically analyze first TMT joint nonunion rates compared with previous reports. We showed a 4% nonunion rate and a 2% revision rate (4 of 201 feet), which is lower than most of the reported nonunions.[28-32] In trying to correlate a lower nonunion rate in comparison to previous studies, we feel adhering to a meticulous operative technique, including preparation of the arthrodesis site, rigid internal fixation with joint compression, strain relief with local bone grafting, tendo-Achilles lengthening (TAL) or gastrocnemius slide for equinus contractures, and postoperative immobilization can help promote fusion of the first TMTJ.

TREATMENT OF TYPE II GRAND RAPIDS ARCH COLLAPSE CLASSIFICATION

Type II GRACC involves forefoot structures and typically displays a hypermobile first ray. Associated findings include hallux valgus, lesser toe deformity, metatarsalgia, and metatarsal stress fractures. The biomechanical failure in this type involves medial column incompetence with weight-bearing transfer to the lesser rays. The authors' preferred surgical treatment includes medial column fusion with first TMT fusion, 1 to 2 intercuneiform fusion, 1 to 2 intermetatarsal fusion. It is not uncommon to have a positive Silverskiold test with type II GRACC, treated with gastrocnemius recession. The 1 to 2 intercuneiform fusion is performed first, and followed by the first TMT fusion. The hallux valgus can be corrected at this stage with positioning of the metatarsal in the appropriate coronal, sagittal, and axial planes and fusion is accomplished with 2 noncannulated screws. A modified McBride and medial metatarsophalangeal joint capsular plication also can be performed to aid in correction of the hallux valgus and help prevent recurrence.

TREATMENT OF TYPE III GRAND RAPIDS ARCH COLLAPSE CLASSIFICATION

Type III GRACC involves the midfoot with development of midfoot arthritis in the second and third TMT joints (**Fig. 10**). Medial navicular arthritis also may be present, but the biomechanical failure is transverse arch collapse. Arch collapse occurs as a result of medial column collapse and the stress of weight bearing is transferred to the second and third rays; more specifically, the dorsal side of the joints. Because the second TMT, third TMT, and/or NC joints are arthritic, pain improvement and arch reconstruction is successfully treated with a combination of fusions ranging from first and second TMT fusions to first through third TMT with NC fusion (**Fig. 11**).

TREATMENT OF TYPE IV GRAND RAPIDS ARCH COLLAPSE CLASSIFICATION

Elevation of the first ray can produce spring ligament attenuation leading to lateral or dorsolateral peritalar subluxation and subsequent hindfoot valgus deformity. This hindfoot valgus pathology is the defining characteristic of the Grand Rapids type IV deformity, which can be flexible or rigid, based on subtalar motion. A Grand Rapids type IV would also display PTTD, sinus tarsi impingement, and lateral hindfoot/

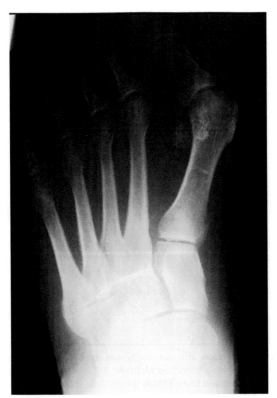

Fig. 10. Anterior to posterior X-ray of foot showing midfoot compression, representing GRACC Type 3. Notice compression at the second and third tarsometatarsal joints.

subtalar arthritis; all of which occur with increasing hindfoot valgus associated with spring ligament attenuation and uncovering of the talar head, which allows for divergence of the talocalcaneal angle and further elevation of the first ray. For comparison, the type IV GRACC would include components of Johnson stage IIB, with talonavicular uncoverage, up to stage IV, with rigid hindfoot valgus. The optimal treatment in this stage is highly dependent on physical examination findings and evidence of talonavicular or subtalar arthritis (**Figs. 1, 12** and **13**).

Type IV GRACC hindfoot valgus can be corrected with a calcaneal osteotomy in flexible deformities, or the inclusion of subtalar and/or talonavicular arthrodesis when these joints are arthritic. Corrections also can include triple arthrodesis of the subtalar, talonavicular, and calcaneocuboid joints. Because the spring ligament is attenuated, a repair can be used in flexible deformities but is unnecessary when fusion is performed, at least across the talonavicular joint. The diseased PTT may be debrided, if minimal tendinosis present, or excised, when severe tendinosis and scarring are present. Controversy does exist with respect to whether or not to excise or retain the PTT when there is a functional tendon with associated areas of tendinosis or large chronic but repairable tear or tears. One school of thought is that the diseased PTT is a pain generator that will likely cause persistent discomfort if maintained. The other school of thought is that the PTT is stronger than the muscle tendon used to replace it, and therefore it would biomechanically make sense to preserve it.[33]

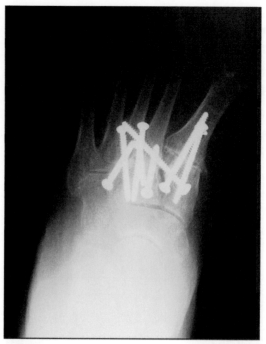

Fig. 11. GRACC type III correction. This deformity was corrected with a gastrocnemius recession, first TMT arthrodesis with a modified McBride, 1-2 intermetatarsal and 1-2 intercuneiform arthrodesis, and second and third TMT arthrodesis to treat the midfoot pain/instability.

The rigid arthritic hindfoot with PTTD has traditionally been completed with a dual incision triple or double arthrodesis. Ryerson[34] first described this dual incision technique in 1923 as treatment of a rigid deformity secondary to paralytic conditions. However, as these types of diseases became less common, the triple arthrodesis was used to correct rigid arthritic adult flatfoot.[35,36] This procedure would be contraindicated in patients with poor soft tissue or poor vascular status of the hindfoot. In all of the type III and type IV deformities, treatment of the hallux valgus is still the same, as it would be in type II deformities, with restoration of coronal, sagittal, and rotational deformity of the

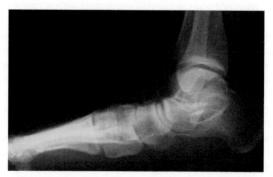

Fig. 12. Weight-bearing lateral radiograph view of flatfoot collapse (type IV GRACC). The progression to involvement of the hindfoot is a hallmark of type IV GRACC.

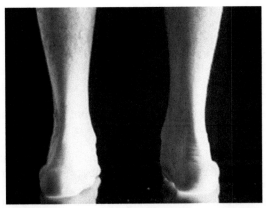

Fig. 13. Anatomic demonstration of flatfoot collapse (type IV GRACC). The left side displays hindfoot valgus while the right side shows neutral alignment.

first ray. Type III and IV deformities, which by nature entail additional deformities in the midfoot or hindfoot, will typically require more extensive reconstruction of the midfoot joints or hindfoot. This depends on where the deformity extends proximal to the forefoot.

SUMMARY

As we evaluate patients with PTTD and arch collapse, we must stabilize and correct the deformities with the understanding of failure in 3 dimensions. Historically, bunions have focused on the coronal plane; however, as we discussed earlier, there is tension and compression failure in the sagittal plane of the midfoot during arch collapse. Correction of all 3 planes of deformity, coronal, sagittal, and rotational, can be achieved in several ways. Some investigators prefer a combination of osteotomies to the first metatarsal. We have shown TMT fusion (96+% fusion rate) with 1 to 2 inter-metatarsal and 1 to 2 intercuneiform fusions to be a reliable way to correct these deformities, stabilize the first ray and maintain arch support, prevent transfer lesions, and have recently demonstrated the potential for early weight bearing postoperatively. Taking a big picture of global foot mechanics by recognizing the common types of conditions associated with arch collapse, including hallux valgus deformities, can serve as a useful roadmap for navigating more complicated deformities where hallux valgus exists.

ACKNOWLEDGEMENTS

The authors would like to acknowledge Dr. John Anderson and Dr. Donald Bohay for their contributions to this chapter.

REFERENCES

1. Gould N, Scheider S, Ashikaga T. Epidemiologic survey of foot problems in the continental United States: 1978-9. Foot Ankle 1980;1:8–10.
2. Johnson KA, Strom DE. Tibialis posterior tendon dysfunction. Clin Orthop Relat Res 1989;239:196–206.
3. Van Boerum DH, Sangeorzan BJ. Biomechanics and pathophysiology of flat foot. Foot Ankle Clin 2003;8:419–30.

4. Lapidus PW. Kinesiology and mechanical anatomy of the tarsal joints. Clin Orthop Relat Res 1963;30:20–36.

5. DiGiovanni CW, Kuo R, Tejwani N, et al. Isolated gastrocnemius tightness. J Bone Joint Surg Am 2002;84:962–70.

6. Coetzee JC, Castro MD. The indications and biomechanical rationale for various hindfoot procedure in the treatment of posterior tibial tendon dysfunction. Foot Ankle Clin 2003;8:453–9.

7. Hicks JH. The mechanics of the foot. II. The plantar aponeurosis and the arch. J Anat 1954;88:25–30.

8. Cotton FJ. Foot statics and surgery. N Engl J Med 1936;214:353–62.

9. Singh D, Biz C, Corradin M, et al. Comparison of dorsal and dorsomedial displacement in evaluation of first ray hypermobility in feet with and without hallux valgus. Foot Ankle Surg 2016;22(2):120–4.

10. Taylor NG, Metcalfe SA. A review of surgical outcomes of the Lapidus procedure for treatment of hallux abductovalgus and degenerative joint disease of the first MCJ. Foot (Edinb) 2008;18(4):206–10.

11. Anderson JG, Hansen ST. Surgical treatment of posterior tendon pathology. In: Kelikien AS, editor. Operative treatment of the foot and ankle. Standford (CT): Appleton & Lange; 1999. p. 211–3.

12. Habbu R, Holthusen SM, Anderson JG, et al. Operative correction of arch collapse with forefoot deformity: a retrospective analysis of outcomes. Foot Ankle Int 2011;32(8):764–73.

13. Eustace S, Byrne JO, Beausang O, et al. Hallux valgus, first metatarsal pronation and collapse of the medial longitudinal arch–a radiological correlation. Skeletal Radiol 1994;23(3):191–4.

14. Dayton P, Feilmeier M, Kauwe M, et al. Relationship of frontal plane rotation of first metatarsal to proximal articular set angle and hallux alignment in patients undergoing tarsometatarsal arthrodesis for hallux abducto valgus: a case series and critical review of the literature. J Foot Ankle Surg 2013;52(3):348–54.

15. Kaplan EB. The tibialis posterior muscle in relation to hallux valgus. Bull Hosp Joint Dis 1955;16:88–93.

16. Gunal I, Sahinoglu K, Bergman RDA. Anomalous tibialis posterior muscle as an etiologic factor of hallux valgus. Clin Anat 1994;7:21–5.

17. Wong YS. Influence of the abductor hallucis muscle on the medial arch of the foot: a kinematic and anatomical cadaver study. Foot Ankle Int 2007;28(5): 617–20.

18. Willegger M, Holinka J, Ristl R, et al. Correction power and complications of first tarsometatarsal joint arthrodesis for hallux valgus deformity. Int Orthop 2015; 39(3):467–76.

19. Peterson KS, McAlister JE, Hyer CF, et al. Symptomatic hardware removal after first tarsometatarsal arthrodesis. J Foot Ankle Surg 2016;55(1):55–9.

20. Shibuya N, Roukis TS, Jupiter DC. Mobility of the first ray in patients with or without hallux valgus deformity: systematic review and meta-analysis. J Foot Ankle Surg 2017;56(5):1070–5.

21. Mani SB, Lloyd EW, MacMahon A, et al. Modified Lapidus procedure with joint compression, meticulous surface preparation, and shear-strain-relieved bone graft yields low nonunion rate. HSS J 2015;11(3):243–8.

22. Barp EA, Erickson JG, Smith HL, et al. Evaluation of fixation techniques for meta-tarsocuneiform arthrodesis. J Foot Ankle Surg 2017;56(3):468–73.

23. Donnenwerth MP, Borkosky SL, Abicht BP, et al. Rate of nonunion after first metatarsal-cuneiform arthrodesis using joint curettage and two crossed

compression screw fixation: a systematic review. J Foot Ankle Surg 2011;50(6): 707–9.

24. King CM, Richey J, Patel S, et al. Modified Lapidus arthrodesis with crossed screw fixation: early weightbearing in 136 patients. J Foot Ankle Surg 2015; 54(1):69–75.

25. Gutteck N, Wohlrab D, Zeh A, et al. Immediate full weightbearing after tarsometatarsal arthrodesis for hallux valgus correction—does it increase the complication rate? Foot Ankle Surg 2015;21(3):198–201.

26. Kazzaz S, Singh D. Postoperative cast necessity after a lapidus arthrodesis. Foot Ankle Int 2009;30(8):746–51.

27. MacMahon A, Karbassi J, Burket JC, et al. Return to sports and physical activities after the modified Lapidus procedure for hallux valgus in young patients. Foot Ankle Int 2016;37(4):378–85.

28. Mauldin DM, Sanders M, Whitmer WW. Correction of hallux valgus with metatarso-cuneiform stabilization. Foot Ankle 1990;11:59–66.

29. Myerson M, Allon S, McGarvey W. Metatarso-cuneiform arthrodesis for management of hallux valgus and metatarsus primus varus. Foot Ankle 1998;13:376–85.

30. Saffo G, Wooster MF, Stevens M, et al. First metatarsocuneiform arthrodesis: a five-year retrospective analysis. J Foot Surg 1989;28:459–63.

31. Sangeorzan B, Hansen ST Jr. Modified Lapidus procedure for hallux valgus. Foot Ankle 1989;9:262–6.

32. Catanzariti A, Mendicino RW, Lee MS, et al. The modified Lapidus arthrodesis: retrospective analysis. J Foot Ankle Surg 1999;38:322–32.

33. Raikin S, Myerson M. Adult flatfoot. Foot Ankle Clin N Am 2012;17(2):205–27.

34. Ryerson E. Arthrodesing operations on the feet. J Bone Joint Surg Am 1923;5: 453–71.

35. Wilson FC Jr, Fay GF, Lamotte P, et al. Triple arthrodesis: a study of the factors affecting fusion after three hundred and one procedures. J Bone Joint Surg Am 1965;47:340–8.

36. Duncan LW, Lovell WW. Hoke triple arthrodesis. J Bone Joint Surg Am 1978;60: 796–8.

Moving?

Make sure your subscription moves with you!

To notify us of your new address, find your **Clinics Account Number** (located on your mailing label above your name), and contact customer service at:

Email: journalscustomerservice-usa@elsevier.com

800-654-2452 (subscribers in the U.S. & Canada)
314-447-8871 (subscribers outside of the U.S. & Canada)

Fax number: 314-447-8029

Elsevier Health Sciences Division
Subscription Customer Service
3251 Riverport Lane
Maryland Heights, MO 63043

*To ensure uninterrupted delivery of your subscription, please notify us at least 4 weeks in advance of move.

Printed and bound by CPI Group (UK) Ltd, Croydon, CR0 4YY

08/05/2025

01864713-0005